Delicious
Healing

Dr. Tumi Johnson, M.D.

BALBOA.PRESS
A DIVISION OF HAY HOUSE

Balboa Press books may be ordered through booksellers or by contacting:

Balboa Press
A Division of Hay House
1663 Liberty Drive
Bloomington, IN 47403
www.balboapress.com
1 (877) 407-4847

Print information available on the last page.

ISBN: 978-1-5043-9427-7 (sc)
ISBN: 978-1-5043-9428-4 (e)

Library of Congress Control Number: 2017919760

Balboa Press rev. date: 07/21/2020

PATIENT/CLIENT TESTIMONIALS

Dr. Johnson, aka Tumi, is a unique combination of highly skilled MD and holistic practitioner. With her guidance, we seamlessly navigated Western and natural medicine to improve my overall health and well-being. I felt com-fortable speaking with her about all things, both physical and emotional, and our time together helped lay the groundwork for a long-term approach to living well and aging gracefully. What more can I ask for? We even laughed a lot. She is a gift I recommend to anyone who wants to get healthy.

-Rachel M

Dr. Tumi Johnson's holistic medical recommendations have changed my life…I had suffered from constant in-somnia and an inability to lose weight for the last twenty years I was desperate for a good nights sleep. All conventional medical doctors could offer were addictive drugs that worked temporarily but with undesirable side effects.

Her consultations, a home visit and follow up calls were the start of my life improvement and insomnia "cure." Her information and suggestions, were always supported by a gentle "you can do it attitude." With her help and guidance, I was able to make the necessary diet adjustments and some changes to my bedtime routine.

I was surprised that food was related to insomnia, since I was already eating a healthy diet. With her help, guid-ance and continuous encouragement I can sleep through the night and am winning the weight battle.

-Ruby P

Dr. Tumi Johnson is an amazing, brilliant, and compassionate holistic health provider. She is very passionate about natural health and it shows with her providing me with a complete personal plan. She has greatly helped me in my journey to maximize my health.

-Ken L

I feel completely overwhelmed with gratitude and deep joy for what my time with Dr. Tumi Johnson has contrib-uted to my life. From the first time I heard her present at the health festival where we met, I felt moved by her presence. Tumi's intelligence, poise, vast knowledge, compassion, and her desire to serve others by sharing her knowledge and message of full body health have always shined through. Since our first meeting I have had the great pleasure of getting to know Tumi more and she has become the Doctor I always turn to for answers, guid-ance, and the path to reconnect with myself and my health. She has also become a friend, an inspiration, a person I admire deeply for the way she walks this world, sharing her light with all whose paths she crosses. I eagerly recommend Tumi's services to anyone who is interested and I feel confident that your life will be positively changed by your time spent with this truly magnificent being. Thank you, Tumi, for all that you have contributed and continue to bring to my life.

-Brittany T

Tumi's knowledge and unwavering enthusiasm and support was an integral part of my ability to stay with the pro-gram. I appreciated her individualized plan and felt very taken care of by her, as she was genuinely interested in my well-being and overall health. She looks at the whole person, unusual these days. I was comforted by the fact that she is a medical doctor who has gone way beyond what most doctors know of (and are not afraid to admit to). Thank you!

-Linda S

Dr. Johnson is an absolute wealth of information and not only talks the talk but walks the walk! I had been strug-gling with the idea of having to follow the Specific Carbohydrate Diet indefinitely; while it seems to have been helpful for my ulcerative colitis, I was getting increasingly turned off the diet due to its rigidity and limitations. Dr. Johnson has gotten me started down a path that feels like a better fit for me. She also helped me make sense of the often conflicting information out there about how we should be eating. She was extremely available, sup-portive, and professional throughout the process; her sessions are packed with information. Time will tell if this new approach will really help keep my disease under control but so far so good!

-Jane C

Tumi was exactly what my husband and I needed to jump start much needed changes in eating and lifestyle. My husband relies on evidence when making decisions and I tend to feel motivated by someone's strong conviction and support. Tumi provided both, encouraging many significant and healthy changes in our diet while also giving us clear and extensive information to back up why these changes are helpful and important. An additional bonus to doing this work has been that my husband and I have a much better time planning for and preparing meals, especially since we're both in the same boat. We also feel so much better than we did one month ago and have steadily lost unwanted weight. THANK YOU TUMI!

-Katie M

Dr. Tumi helped me to achieve a health plan that worked for me. I had tried to incorporate more yoga and medita-tion and a plant based diet into my life previously, but it always seemed too daunting or not worth it in the end. I would always start things only to get discouraged and not follow through. Working with Tumi took the mystery and frustration out of the process and helped me to find a rhythm that I could stick with. Tumi always reminded me that this is a lifestyle change and that a little "mistake" here and there is no reason to give up on positive change. I am so happy with how I am treating my body and I look forward to growing within this practice to con-tinue to strengthen my body and mind. There is definitely a long road ahead to wellness, but I feel confident that I have enough experience, through Tumi's guidance to sustain this for my entire life.

- Anna M

I initially contacted Dr. Tumi to help me implement a plan for my inguinal hernia and high blood pressure. From our first consult, I was immediately blown away by the ease I felt, the feeling of safety, reassurance, and knowledge that she was in it wholly for my best interest. Her expertise in various fields of healing was immense. I never once felt rushed or unheard. She took the time to answer all my questions and then some. I came away learning so much more about my health and dietary choices, and how I can better my mind, body and spirit. I learned to step back and quiet my mind and be empowered to think about what foods I am putting into my body. I am convinced Dr. Tumi sees the whole potential of her patients and doesn't just treat the symptoms by giving quick pills and fixes.

She delved into to the heart of each problem I lay before her and adeptly recommended real-istic and effective strategies to overcome each problem. Dr. Tumi is unlike any doctor or medical professional I have worked with in the past. Her attention to detail, drawing from many areas of western and holistic medicine, and genuine compassion for her patients is evident and places her above all the rest in my opinion. She has given me new hope to pick myself up, when I was down.

Since the initial consultation with Dr. Tumi, I have had the pleasure of several more sessions with her and every time I experienced and learning something new. If I had to describe it in a sentence, I would have to say it was like having a visit with a western medical doctor, a holistic doctor, cognitive therapist and health/wellness coach all rolled into one person! I was pleased that she worked with my local naturopath and was able to receive my bloodwork and interpret the results with me. I like her philosophy in knowing that the body can heal itself if it has the right nutrients and dietary fuel. I cannot recommend Dr. Tumi enough or sing enough praises about my experience and only hope more people will seek out her expertise to help them overcome their health and well-ness concerns. She is a rare gem who is doing so much for the betterment of humanity and ultimately the well-ness of our planet.

- Jason N

* to read more client testimonials please
visit www.drtumijohnson.com *

ABOUT THE AUTHOR

Dr. Oluwatumininu (Tumi) Johnson, M.D. is a physician, dancer, and poet.

She is board certified in Internal Medicine, a diplomate of the American Board of Integrative Holistic Medicine, and became an Assistant Clinical Professor of Medicine at NYU in 2011. She has been a yoga practitioner for over 20 years and completed Yoga teacher training with Yogaworks in 2012. A graduate of the Institute of Integrative Nutrition, Dr. Johnson also has extensive nutrition expertise, with past experience running a weight management clinic in New York City. Tumi also served in West Africa as a Doctors Without Borders field doctor in nutrition clinics there.

Her holistic medical practice is focused on helping people identify the underlying causes of their health issues. She then uses her expertise to offer individualized holistic regimens that support people in achieving and sustaining their most vibrant well-being. Through her plant-based health plans, she has had many patients heal issues ranging from diabetes to hormonal imbalances to persistent weight challenges.

As a dancer, Dr. Johnson creates and performs dance pieces crafted from original poetry, that are intended to help the healing process of those who witness the dance. Her dances have been performed in southern France, Haiti, West Africa, Asia, and throughout the U.S.

Dr. Johnson is dedicated to empowering others in their journeys of personal health, peace, and happiness, and this book is written with that intention. She offers her story to help dismantle the shame of the many who go through trauma and disease, often self-inflicted, as a testament that often our deepest wounds can be our greatest gifts not just to ourselves but also to others. She writes this book so that people will witness that even those "who know better," medical professionals, can fall victim to disease-causing habits. This book is the doctor's white coat being taken off in a way that she hopes to be healing for anyone who mistakenly views physicians as super human or maybe even inhuman. As both doctor and poet-dancer, through this book, she provides a creative and unique mix of practical, science-based advice blended with art (through poetry and dance). This blend reaches the heart and can motivate and transform in a way that just the facts never can. More than anything else, this book is offered in love, the most powerful healer of all.

drtumijohnson.com

Instagram/YouTube: thepoemdances

CONTENTS

About the Author xi
Introduction: Physician, heal thyself xvii
Before Diving in: Intention setting and Visualization xxiii

Chapter 1   Delicious Food As Thy Medicine 1
Chapter 2   Your Movement practice 19
Chapter 3   Meditation/Mindfulness 37
Chapter 4   Sleep and Rest 53
Chapter 5   Emotion honoring and release 73
Chapter 6   Nature 89
Chapter 7   Love 105

References 123
Acknowledgments 129

Dedicated to you.

INTRODUCTION

Physician, heal thyself

Renaissance

After she swallowed the pill, the girl thought—
I wish it were the sugar-coated kind I'd bought.
I had forgotten how bitter these can be.
Finishing fifty will take an eternity.
But then she thought—well I shall have that long;
I just wish to help me through, I had a song.
She was sitting in the antechamber of an old church
where no one would have searched.
It was midnight, a Friday in January
and being found would be unlikely.
So she took her time with the sour tablets
but on the fifteenth swallow, began to fret.
It was cold, the smell was making her ill
and she was unsure thirty five would seal the deal.
She found a sweater in her sack, wore it.
The shivers subsided but she wished the hall lit.
Twenty one, twenty two, halfway through, she began to falter,
not from fear. The pills were sticking. She wished for water.
At pill thirty, she thought—shit, I shall die a virgin
and it won't even be enough to pardon this sin.
And if I begin to see visions, it won't be Gabriel
but Lucifer's warden with a two-pronged tail.
She laughed at pill thirty, there were tears as well,
then gagged from the taste and smell.
On the fortieth, she thought—they will cry
but mostly they will hate me, not ask "Why?"

Rapidly, she took three more
and rested her head on the hardwood floor.

N-acetylcysteine was given to save her liver.
Her family was around her, she broke her fever.
On the fourth day, she awoke to find herself alone,
a blank paged silence took the room. But no.
A figure was sitting at the foot of the bed
and finally, she was she certain she must be dead.
"Did my liver finally give out?"
No answer, then with a turn and a shout,
"Ah, but I how I love Millay!"
The girl stared. The woman had her eyes, her nose looked the
same way.
But her hair was thicker, and how her skin glowed.
"Are you God?" she asked, but then she saw the clothes.
The red dip of décolletage. The woman put the poetry down.
Her fingernails were multicolored. The girl frowned.
"I would never, ever wear those colors."
"Maybe that's your problem. They are only colors."
She smiled. She was beautiful. The girl began to cry.
"To live this life feels harder than to die.
I think there's something wrong with my brain."
"It's true. You are different, strange, it's plain."
"I have no idea what to do."
"Do whatever works for you."
"I've tried. Prayer, yoga. I drink green tea."
"Stay in bhujangasana longer than you care to be.
Pray for what you truly desire
and wear color, it'll keep your soul afire
because if the soul is flat…"
She pushed her hair back.
She tucked the poem under her arm and leaned in,
"Remember heaven is amidst strangeness, amidst sin and kin."

From the top of her breast, a new birthmark climbed into view.
"Just write the song that gets you through."

-Tumi Johnson

I was about 23 when the above happened. A near death experience
is often described in hindsight by those who have gone through it,
as a life changing occurrence. I feel no different. Maybe there is
something about it that jolts one out of complacency. Something
that makes one re-examine just what one is doing with one's life
when that life is returned to you after being a hair's breath away
from losing it. Especially when it is you that almost gave it away. I
was about 23 years old, a young woman from a good family, doing
well academically at a great medical school, with wonderful friends.
When my sister brought me to the ER after my suicide attempt,
the nurse took a look at my chart and then at my face and said
"But honey, you're too pretty to do something like this." I had what
seemed like everything going for me. However, it's a cliché for a
reason: looks can be deceiving. I was a physician-in-training in deep
need of healing.

Among my health issues were a life-long struggle with asthma, a
more recent struggle with disordered eating that began around the
time of the dissolution of my parent's marriage, and depression that
could put me in what felt like a haze, for days on end. I was a dancer
who wasn't dancing enough, I was a daughter too frightened to speak
her truth. I was a woman that felt disempowered in many realms
of her life. I was experiencing a real disconnect between the life I
desired and the life I felt I was barely living. At some point in that
hospital bed, I made a pact with God. I looked out and saw a female
resident physician making her evening rounds and I experienced a
powerful clench in my mid-section. It was at that very moment I
understood how much I wanted to be a doctor. And so I prayed,
"please let me live so I can be who I truly want to be." I didn't yet

understand the power of those words and it took me years to unpack the tangle of dis-eases I listed above, to arrive here. And "here" is the other side of the suffering. And it is from here that I write to you and say that my renaissance, my "rebirth," began, as it often does, with a feeling of brokenness and utter powerlessness. But that space is a curious one, isn't it? Because from there, all pretense and ego fall away, and you can lift up your truest prayer. And witness magic begin to occur.

This book is the practical "breakdown" of that magic, the components of which were vital to my healing. They are the tools that I used and honed over the next several years to create and joyfully live my very best life, as I do now. They are the tools that I share with those I am privileged to work with. I share them here with you in the hopes that you feel empowered to create with greater ease, your most vibrant and healthy existence. May it be so.

BEFORE DIVING IN

Intention setting and Visualization

Cormorant Anthem

I was called greedy
when they saw my wingspan.
Antinomian. I stretched out
wide arms and rose for flight. I craned my neck.
I took my fill. They called me the devil.
But they were absent at the prelude.

I had to train myself to give up this weight.
I vomited before predators came, to be sharper for the fight, lighter for the flight.
I had to show that this sleeve of fear was disposable. I needed nothing
physical, no burdens, no thing. They thought me vulgar
when I unzipped my dress and dove into dance.
But they did not know me at the start, when
I was something more inchoate, those
moments my head bent to a gaze,
the shame at my bill's curve.
Now my mouth is a
blade. I need no
pretty songs
when I
fill the
sky.

-Tumi Johnson

When I meet with a patient or client for the first time, the first thing
I ask is NOT what they are eating. I don't do a 24 hr diet recall (yet)
nor collect a food diary. I am a huge proponent of the fact that food
is our medicine and that what we choose to put and *not* put into

our bodies can absolutely transform our lives for the better or worse. However, there is something even more powerful than issues around food, in making and sustaining positive changes in your health. And that is your intention. The first thing I ask is "What do you want?" "What life do you want to create?" "What sort of health do you want to make into a reality?" What I have witnessed is that the level of clarity of the answer to these questions is often a foreshadowing of what is to come. In short, if all you can see is a life of one health problem after the other, that is often what you'll get. If however, you can put aside limiting beliefs of what is possible or what you have (up until now) experienced, close your eyes and imagine the health you want to create, you begin to tap into a power that has the potential to make that dream a reality.

There is a well-known quote that states "when the student is ready, the teacher will appear." I would add to this by saying that if the student is not ready, the teacher might be in plain sight, hopping on one foot and waving both arms, and the student will not see him or her. Ever since I began my holistic medical practice, I have noticed something quite interesting. And it is the difference between people who approach me on their own (including those who have received recommendations about me from others) and those who approach me because they have been "gifted" a session with me by someone, but who otherwise wouldn't have sought out guidance. People who initiate work with me have an answer when I ask "what life do you want to create?" are a joy to work with and there are always rapid and positive health shifts when we start working together. With those who come to the first session because someone else made it too easy to say no, the result is often less consistent.

To see powerful and sustained positive changes in your health, I strongly recommend to first dream. Dream of what it looks like to have your best life. What do you look like? Where do you live? What are you doing? Who are you doing it with? I say this because almost always, when I ask people what they want and they *do* give me a clear answer, I am still surprised by how humble those answers are. "Losing fifteen pounds" (when they'd really like to lose thirty), "to have less pain" (when they'd prefer *no* pain), or "to find natural ways of treating my uterine fibroids" when the true secret dream is to have a healthy uterus and be able to carry and healthily birth a chid with ease.

And yet I shouldn't be surprised with the answers I often hear. We have almost all witnessed medical institutions that have let us down over and over again in terms of failed promises and sometimes worse, harm, rather than healing, being done. We have gotten used to rushed fifteen minute visits with doctors so that people feel they have to minimize their health requests and get those requests out of their mouths as quickly as possible. We are used to a "health" establishment that is actually a sick one, focused on sick care, in which if the lingo is not about "treating disease," it's about "preventing disease." But how about not putting the focus on 'disease' but rather on what our bodies' true natural state is— 'vitality,' 'optimal health?' How about speaking on "health promotion" instead of "disease prevention?" One might argue those are the same things but I say not. The latter is limiting, the former is expansive. The former is where your dreams reside.

So practically, what does this look like? How do you dream and get crystal clear about the health you want to create?

Here is….

My Prescription for Intention setting and Visualizing your best health:

1. Take a blank sheet of paper, a writing/drawing instrument and (optional) a musical instrument.

2. Go to a place in nature that you deeply resonate with and fills you with a sense of peace and beauty; ideally choose a spot where you won't be disturbed (at least by fellow humans).

3. Once settled in your spot, ask yourself what your optimally healthy life looks like.

4. Close your eyes, if it is easier for you at this point, as you imagine this life. Stay with the dream as long as it continues to reveal itself to you. Imagine where you are living, who you are living with, how you spend your days, and perhaps most importantly how you FEEL living this life.

5. Play the instrument if you have it then draw anything you are moved to play and/or draw, if that feels good to you.

6. Finally write and/or draw on your paper what you envision your healthy life to be. You might choose to write this in a "day in your best life" format writing how you spend your day from morning to evening. You might choose just to make a list of the feelings or different elements of your healthy life. You might choose to draw these elements of your healthy life. Choose the format you most resonate with.

7. Take this paper home and post it up on your vision board or file it along with your "health documents." This might be the most important health document you have—more than the results of past blood tests or health insurance bills, because it is a statement of your desired well-being, and there is such power in that.

8. The next time you have an appointment with a health care provider (whether it be physical therapist, homeopath, doctor, accupuncturist, etc), bring that piece of paper as important reference for you to return to as you make plans with your health practitioner about your health. Having that paper with you and referring to it routinely will help you stay aligned with your intentions. Also consider sharing its contents with your health care provider. P.S. If your health

care practitioner doesn't approach what this paper that you present with respect and compassion, I strongly recommend you find another.

There are plenty of people in the health care field who are ready to support you in living your best life. With your intentions clearly stated, you are now ready to dive in.

Just a word about navigating the book. Many chapters are bookended with a poem in the beginning and a link to one of my poemdance pieces at the end. I do this to help you emotionally tap into the ideas of the chapter in a way that I feel the arts do beautifully. Feel free to read the poem and watch the dance piece in the order they are presented or before or after reading the written chapter content itself. Do whatever resonates most with you; you will hear that invitation a lot during reading this book. Also, as was introduced with this very chapter you are reading, there will be a prescription at the end of each following chapter. It's usually a practical exercise to help you implement the ideas of that chapter into your very individual life. Please try them out. I recommend having a blank journal and using this journal to do these offered exercises in "real time," at the end of each chapter. However, if you feel more like just reading the book through once, then going back and doing each of the chapter prescriptions after your first read-through, that is a great alternative way to go through this book. Okay, enough prep. Are you ready? Please read on for my offered seven vital components to having a delicious and healthy life.

CHAPTER 1

Delicious Food As Thy Medicine

Durian Haiku

Crack the spiked armor
take in its waft of sweet stink
delight in the cream

- Tumi Johnson

There is a reason I am beginning these chapters with the one on food. In my personal and clinical experience, a healthy diet— one that truly supports your most vibrant well-being is foundational for one's best life. And it is often an aspect of people's health that is in need of great help. There are many people who clean up their diet after a spiritual or emotional awakening but I think one of the easiest ways to "level up" emotionally, mentally, as well as physically, is to level up one's diet.

Easier said than done, one might say. There is a reason why diet books are a multi-million dollar industry. And the plethora of health problems that come with poor nutrition is not just limited to the "Western world." Thanks in part to the McDonaldization of the globe (and I mean this in the literal sense, not necessarily George Ritzer's definition [1]), type II diabetes, obesity, heart disease, and cancer are growing at disturbing rates all over the world. I hear so often now when I'm in a country in Asia or Africa: "I was here a few years ago and there were not this amount of overweight people." Even the French are getting fat, though they have a secret that I will share a little later on that works very well for keeping slim and healthy.

Dr. Tumi Johnson, M.D.

As I was writing this chapter in my apartment in Chiang Mai, Thailand, I thought "Is it too easy to blame this on McDonalds?" and then I looked through my window and saw a huge red sign with the famous golden arches. A sign that was not there a year ago when I occupied this same living space.

Sometimes the right answers are the simplest ones. What I have witnessed over and over in medical clinical work is that the further away people are eating from a natural, whole foods diet, the sicker they are. Especially when they are eating a lot of it. And the funny thing about processed and "refined" food (such a misnomer— there is nothing refined about a Twinkie): it is very easy to eat a lot of it. A few years back, I was car-pooling in Southern California with a friend, heading from Ojai to Carlsbad for an awards ceremony. We were in central L.A. when she realized that she had to do some urgent work that needed to be submitted online within the next two hours. The only place we could find in the neighborhood was a well known fast food chain restaurant (cough "golden arches"). It had been years since I'd been in this place and literally the only thing I felt comfortable ordering was hot water. This specific branch didn't even have non-caffeinated tea. So I sat cradling my hot water (it was a strangely cool morning) and while she worked, I looked around. There was the familiar ubiquitous children's play area and plenty of shiny seats. Over the next ninety minutes as my friend frantically completed her work, I noted something that was at best alarming and perhaps even sinister. I watched children (from ages five to about eleven years old) come in with their parents and order fast food. Some left within five minutes of eating their meal, but for anyone who stayed longer than fifteen minutes after their meal, the children who for the most case, had been calm, became extremely agitated. I have a good amount of experience with children, and this response was not about boredom. They became nervous and angry. It was like clockwork and I was riveted to it all. At some point, the parents would take them to the indoor jungle gym which sometimes

4

helped and sometimes not and then finally, the child was shuttled out of the place. When a grown young man (probably early 20s) who had been silently eating in the corner all by himself and who I had ignored up until now, let out an angry prolonged shout for no apparent reason, I decided it was time for me to go. Thankfully, my friend was putting the last touches on her work and we left very soon after. Now that was one branch of one fast food chain and just a ninety minute snippet at that, but it would be an interesting study to look closer at the neuropsychiatric effects on some of these processed foods on our brains, especially those of children. My hypothesis is that it would provide further reason why we should stay very far away from these "foods." But most people know that we should avoid processed food (whether or not it comes from a fast food joint). And apart from the economic reasonings around choosing such foods (processed packaged food usually having a cheap sticker price) and the addictive component of such foods, there is also a physiologic explanation for why it's easy to over-do it on processed foods. When you are eating food that is processed, it is often both low in fiber and nutrient poor. The result of that is that you don't get satiated because fiber is quite filling and also because your body, still not having received the nutrients it needs, is still starved even if you are feeding it calories.

For several years, I, like many others, lived this reality. Around the time of my parent's divorce, I began to use food as a way to numb a lot of the very painful emotions that were coming up for me around my parents' relationship and my relationship to them. And "food" is a very loose term for what I was eating. "Drug" is a more apt word and anyone who has eaten compulsively or binged knows that this is not an overstatement. My disordered eating went into full effect soon after starting university. Away from home and yet still heart connected to the painful relationships there, I now had full autonomy to choose my poison. I was away from my mother's home-made pretty healthy meals, and I started eating bagels daily for breakfast. Soon, I began eating them also for lunch and then soon, they became my daily staple for every meal. Sometimes I had this with sweetened soy milk, thinking I was being healthy. Working part time as a coffeeshop barista didn't help my worsening eating habits and soon, a regular lunch for me was a few bagels (not whole-wheat) with a iced OR hot mocha depending on the time of the year. And not surprisingly, I started to put on weight despite being in a dance troupe and working out more regularly than most college students. My punishing exercise regimen and bouts of skipping meals kept me from becoming significantly overweight but I was still carrying more weight than was healthy for my body. Perhaps even more significantly, I had a very disordered relationship with food in which I woke up thinking about how to get the food I wanted, would have then have the food, then having had it, feel numbed out and unable to function until very quickly the gnawing desire for food returned again. It is any wonder I didn't spiral into deep depression and I thank my dance practice and my wonderful group of friends for that. But I remember my low point and that point wasn't a year into this behavior. It was a good four years in, when I steadily ate seven bagels in a bathroom stall, feeling too full after four, almost sick after five but continuing on until I couldn't feel anything. And that's when I had to admit I had a serious problem. Soon, I cut myself off the bread, replacing the diet with an Atkins style regimen (pescetarian style since I'd stopped eating meat except for fish during my early teens). I ate more fish, whenever I could afford to on my student budget, a bit more veggies and lots of dairy and soy, thinking that eating more protein and less carb would be much healthier. And I would feel good, if a bit hungry, until a brief binge episode on bread or packaged cereal or some other processed high carb food. I would then repent to my "good" ways until I was "bad" again. On the outside though, I lost the gained weight, looked like a healthier dancer and was well on my way to graduating from a top university and headed for medical school And yet this drama to which the people in my life (including those closest to me) where clueless to, continued steadily over the next several years. It continued until I wound up in that hospital bed getting medication through an IV to save my liver. Afterwards, I was forced to go through therapy. Appropriately so. And it was in Emily's office (I don't remember her last name, but I'm forever in gratitude), I shared for the first time to anyone about my eating disorder, and began to recover. One of the most powerful things I learned with Emily is that it's not all about the food. I will talk more about the role our emotions play in our health in a later chapter. For now I will just share that recognizing how I was using food to numb emotions, was a vital part of my recovery process.

In this chapter, I will say some of it *is* about the food. It is very hard to numb yourself out on whole fruits and vegetables (much harder than processed foods). That is why if you are an "emotional eater" and use food as a coping mechanism as I did, it is crucial to have an emotion honoring and release practice (more on this in the later chapter). If you don't have this practice, it will be very hard to stay on a healthy, whole foods diet. That said, when you begin replacing processed foods consistently with natural whole foods, your body begins to thrive. Your nutrient levels become replete, your body stops starving and no longer puts out "hunger" cues all the time because it is getting more of what it had been asking for all along. From 2006-2007, I spent nine months in the Tahaoua region of Niger as a Doctors Without Borders' field physician. There, I helped run clinics and hospitals for malnourished children through in part, a re-feeding protocol. One thing I observed during my time there is how incredibly resilient the human being can be, and that when we (even the littlest ones of us) are given the appropriate nutrition, our bodies can fight off the most aggressive of diseases. I watched emaciated children too weak to walk, babies with pregnant looking bellies from kwashiorkor, battling malaria, meningitis, diarrheal illness and cutaneous TB (among many other diseases), transform. They transformed to vibrant children with plump cheeks and eyes that were no longer listless but tracking my every move, after receiving treatment, the cornerstone of which was nutritional support.

After my time as a field doctor in Niger, I returned to my life in New York City. There, I took a good look at myself, much healthier since receiving therapy with much less binging but still not feeling at ease with food. And I had a nagging sensation that my diet was not the most supportive of my best life. I was still battling life-long asthma and eczema, and strong waves of depression still came up routinely, though not like in the past, thanks to a much healthier emotional response practice. It was witnessing the miracles of nutrition during my medical work in West Africa, that motivated me to start looking at how I could improve my own diet. I began more study in the realm of nutrition and long story short, arrived at the simple but powerful and life changing conclusion that a whole foods, plant (and when possible, living) food diet is really how we were designed to eat and that we as a species, thrive on. The evidence that convinced me of the above is extremely rich and broad and beyond the focus of this book. However, I have listed in the bibliography, seminal books, medical studies, and other amazing resources that were incredibly helpful to me in coming to these realizations[2].

What happened to my health after implementing the above was nothing short of astonishing in terms of the complete resolution of my asthma, eczema, severe depression, and just as importantly, my fraught relationship with food. But it wasn't just that I got well. I started to thrive. My dancing got better, my relationship with myself and with others improved and I had an increasingly strong sense of joy, purpose, and peace. That was seven years ago and the journey just continues to get better.

One of the great things about being a doctor is that I get to share knowledge that can make a powerfully positive impact in someone's life, and then watch as it does just that.

I began to ask my patients regularly about their diets. I was (as is typical in most clinics in the U.S.) given 20 minutes per patient during a clinic visit. This is absurd when you're a Primary Care doctor and there are 13 prescriptions written per year per the average American (not including over-the-counter medications, supplements, or herbal medications). But that's a rant for another book. I started using 10 of those 20 minutes to ask people what they were eating and to start counseling on shifting the diet. I began talking to my patients about the importance of eating real, whole food meals that were plant based and as minimally processed as possible (eating apples rather than drinking apple juice or eating a sweet potato rather than french fries, for example). And I began to witness incredible results. Type 2 diabetic patients stopped needing their medications. People with uncontrolled hypertension cut their blood pressure medications from four medications to two to one. Women with PCOS (polycystic ovarian syndrome) stopped needing hormone medications as their body's hormones start balancing, and countless people who had struggled with weight all their lives or after "the babies came," lost the excess weight.

Food is powerful, powerful medicine.

But here is another truth that I have discovered. *How* one eats can be just as powerful as *what* one is eating. I began to have puzzling clients in my holistic practice— men and women who seemed to be doing everything perfectly in their diet, in fact almost "too perfectly;" there was a near neurosis in some of these clients about their knowledge of their macronutrient ratios and their caloric intake. They were getting in great amounts of fruits and vegetables, eating a whole foods, unprocessed diet with very little "cheats" or "treats" (their words) and they didn't feel their best. These were the clients that seemed a little, or a lot, on edge when I met with them, who would pause the longest when I asked them "what's good in your life right now?" This being the case, even when an outsider could point to at least five things that on the surface looked amazing. These were usually the clients who were self-labeled "Type A" personalities and who prided themselves with amazing multi-tasking skills. They were having their power green smoothies with the perfect amount of essential fatty acids and a great big dose of superfoods in them. Yet they were constantly having these smoothies on the run or next to their computers as they worked frenetically to stay ahead of several deadlines. And they couldn't seem to drop those "last 10 pounds" or their HDL cholesterol was stubbornly low, or they were being diagnosed with sluggish thyroids, or everything seemed good on paper but something just "didn't feel right."

This is when I'd like to talk about the French paradox. There have been lots of books written by both the French and those who aren't, sharing theories about the interesting "paradox" of the French eating all the "no-nos"— white bread, heavy meats, cheeses while still managing to stay slim and healthy. Yet their American counterparts on the same diet are getting their first heart attack before the age of 50. The first thing I'll say is that the paradox is a bit of an exaggeration. While living in France, I rented a room from a French lady who was constantly dieting and worried about her weight. And she was not the only one. Also, the "McDonaldization" of the world has not escaped France and one does see more overweight people than before. I think this is in part is due to the declining quality of some of the foods and the rise of the processed fast food industry. I'm probably never going to recommend white bread to anyone but that said, white bread that comes from local, non GMO or pesticide-laden, non hybridized wheat grown in healthy soil and made with good water can taste very differently and induce a healthier response in the body than the hybridized, mono-cropped wheat that comes from depleted soil and is overly refined. The latter, in case it's not clear, is the variety seen overwhelmingly in most American grocery stores. But outside of the food quality differences, I have another explanation for this "French paradox" and it is about *how* the French eat. In all the times I have visited France and during my six months living there, I was always struck by the ceremony around food. I witnessed this at Parisian cafes and restaurants. I also witnessed it in rural southwestern France. There in at roadside bistro in the Dordogne region, I once had lunch and observed a truckload of field workers come in for a meal and spend easily an hour over their food. Throughout the country, I saw a sense of relaxed mindfulness and appreciation about mealtime. This is something that I think is greatly absent in America where meals are taken almost furtively, in the car while driving, while walking, while working on the computer. And then there is the way many Americans speak about food. I don't much hear the French use phrases like "I cheated today" or "I was bad," at least not about food. But in general, many Americans do it constantly. I hear it all the time during client sessions when I ask for a 24 hr diet recall, to review what someone has been eating and to make recommendations. And there is one thing about human nature that I find transcends cultures— if you make something "bad," it takes on a power that's not warranted.

What I am speaking about really is mindfulness. And what I am also speaking about is appreciation. And the two are intimately related. When we take the time to really be with our meals, to focus on what we're eating with presence, there is space for appreciation. And there are studies now that show a link between mindfulness around mealtimes and feeling better satiated, eating less, helping to prevent binge eating tendencies, and achieving healthy weight loss[3-7]. Physiologically, it also makes plenty of sense. If we're eating while in a state of stress, we are eating when our sympathetic nervous system (our fight-or-flight apparatus) is in dominant control. The problem with that is it is our *parasympathetic* system that is in control of digestion. And the parasympathetic system is all about relaxation. Thus, we promote poor digestion if we are eating when stressed. Which is why I don't recommend doing the following activities with eating: driving, walking, watching TV/screen, or working. This can be extremely difficult for some people. I myself used to have a very common habit of eating while watching the screen. However, after I observed and recognized some of the lessons of the "French paradox," I decided to eliminate eating in front of the computer screen (I don't own a TV) and practice mindful eating. It took me over six months to do it successfully. And what I learned during those six months was that mindless eating was serving a purpose for me. It was part of my "numbing out" process; it was part of me not facing or acknowledging my emotions. Which is why I have devoted a whole chapter to this issue (coming up). For you, it may take you a couple of days to move to just mindful eating but if you find that there is an emotional reason for eating in a purposefully distracted manner, I think you'll find Chapter 5 especially useful.

Once I started consistently eating mindfully, it was amazing what unfolded. I started making better choices about *what* I ate. I also didn't need as much food. This is likely partly due to the fact that mindful eating also means slower eating which allows for your body to know the moment it's had enough. But also, if you're eating while relaxed and present, you are digesting better which means better assimilation of your nutrients and that translates to not needing as much quantity of food. This has been my experience and afterwards, the experience of many of my clients and patients with whom I share this (I couldn't keep the secret a secret nor would I want to!) So what I advise now is eat mindfully. Each time you eat, even it's just for 10 minutes (you might be saying, "I don't live in a place where I can have relaxed one hour lunches"). No matter how long you have to eat, do it with a sense of presence and appreciation. This can be helped by a moment of gratitude for your meal — where it came from, who grew its components, etc. and if it resonates with you, a prayer of thankfulness. When you take that moment to give thanks for your meal, you'll find it gets harder and harder to eat crappy food because it can be hard to say "thank you" over highly processed/junk food.

There is something also that occurs when you start consistently making healthier choices around food, when you move towards a diet abundant in fresh fruits and vegetables, Nature's offerings. Your palate changes. It is a beautiful moment when you can enjoy a fresh peach unencumbered by anything else and taste the subtle differences in fragrance, texture, and flavor, from one peach to the next. This change bespeaks of a sensory system that is more fine-tuned and sensitive and in turn, an organism that is the same. I am never bored by a bowl of plums as a meal because each is its own slightly different world and it is a pleasure to explore each one.

Which leads me to my final but hugely important point of this chapter. There is real misunderstanding around healthy food and how it tastes. There is a nasty, self-sabotaging, and very false idea circulating around that if something is good for you, it can't possibly taste very good. People talk about eating an apple when they "are being good" but indulging in donuts as a "treat." My common response to that is "how much of a treat do those donuts feel like the next morning when you feel bloated or even just hours later during a sugar crash?" My idea of a real treat (food-wise) is something that tastes delicious when I'm eating it AND which helps me feel (and look) my best afterwards. There are more and more celebrated chefs who are dispelling the idea that fruits and vegetables are boring but frankly, you don't need to go to a Michelin- starred restaurant to discover that. Mother Nature is pretty democratic. Go apple picking in the autumn, enjoy any ripe, fresh, organic fruit in season and enjoy the sound of tumbling walls as the idea of un-tasty healthy food comes crashing down. Biologically, evolutionarily, it makes no sense that the food we are designed to eat, in its unprocessed state, wouldn't taste good to us. I repeat that, *in its unprocessed state*. Please don't think that because chocolate chip cookies taste good to you, I am saying that we are designed to eat them. If you take away the "refining" process, the adding this and extracting that, the cooking of the food in question, and you are left with the food as Mother

Nature presents it to you its true natural state, would you find it enjoyable? If not, I would reconsider it as a food you should be eating on the regular. There are two main reasons why unprocessed natural healthy food might not taste good to you. The first reason is that you are eating these natural foods when they aren't fresh and specifically in the case of fruits, when they are unripe. I have had patients, clients, friends and some family members swear up and down to me that they didn't like fruit but upon further investigation, it was clear that the fruit they found "tasteless" or "yucky" that they had sampled, hadn't been ripe. It is standard practice in many grocery stores (especially large ones) to have fruit that is picked from the tree *before* it is ripe and sold in an underripe state. If you want to truly decide that you don't like a fruit, first make sure that you are eating it when ripe (and preferably tree-ripened). If you are not privy to a fruit tree in your backyard, then try fruit picking at a nearby orchard if that's available to you and select the fruit that easily comes from the tree or even better, the one the tree just 'hands' to you...fruit that has just fallen from its branches. *These* are ripe fruit and it's rare to find them at most grocery stores. The other option which I do often (while I wait for my own fruit trees to grow) is to visit your local farmers' market if that is available to you. Talk to the fruit seller and ask which of the fruits are the most ripe and most freshly picked. One of the many great things about most farmers' markets apart from being able to talk to and thank those who have grown your food, is that the produce is usually quite fresh (newly harvested). Also, start getting comfortable with handling (gently) the fruit yourself. Most ripe fruit in general will have a lovely (but not fermented) slight fragrance, and there will be a slight give to them; in the case of Hachiya persimmons, for example, there needs to be a lot of give to them. Just start practicing and you will learn. There are also some great sources that contain tips on picking ripe fruit as well as knowing which fruit you can pick that might be underripe but that you can ripen at home, if needed. Again, this is less ideal than tree-ripened fruit but that is not always something to which we all have access. I cannot over-emphasize the importance of ripeness as an important factor when picking fruit as well as freshness when selecting fruits and vegetables. These two qualities apart from revealing the accurate tastiness of the food, also reflect the nutrition of the food in question. Un-fresh and un-ripe fruit has less bio-available nutrients than produce that is both fresh and ripe. Again, Mother Nature having our backs.

The second reason why unprocessed natural healthy food might not taste good to you goes back to a statement I mentioned earlier about palate. Your taste buds may have been hijacked (through sensory overload) by years of eating processed foods. These foods contain lots of preservatives and additives (maybe including flavor "enhancers" like MSG), that can erode the appreciation for the natural flavors that your body was designed to enjoy. I have found in my clinical experience that a detox period in which processed foods are completely eliminated helps tremendously in "reviving" our palates so that they can experience both "healthy" and "delicious" in the same bite, just as it was intended to be.

I think pleasure is something that is absent in many of our food experiences. And I'm not talking about pleasure that feels "stolen" or rimmed with guilt or shame about "being bad." Rather, I am speaking about an innocent and open-hearted joy that comes when we are eating food that pleases our eyes and mouth, and also nourishes us physically and mentally. This is what occurs when we are eating real food with which we co-evolved, that is the best fuel for our bodies.

These days, I usually eat just twice a day without any snacks but when I do have those meals whether it's a fifteen minute episode or a ninety minute languorous affair shared with loved ones, I do it with such gratitude. Gratitude for being able to eat and enjoy eating, free of neurosis or the itchy feeling of food addiction. Gratitude for those who have grown the food and if it's applicable, prepared it for me. Gratitude for Divine wisdom in creating such delicious food that also supports my best health (what kindness). Gratitude for Mama Earth's abundance and generosity. Gratitude for the taste of it and being able to enjoy these tastes with someone I love (and sometimes that someone is just me). It is a beautiful and life-affirming way to eat and I hope that some of what I have shared with you during this chapter helps to heal your relationship with food (and with yourself) if needed. May it help clear your path to eating and living deliciously and healthfully.

My Prescription for eating deliciously and healthfully (A Mindful Eating exercise):

> *"I have eaten/the plums/that were in/the icebox and which/you were probably/saving/for breakfast. Forgive me/they were so delicious/so sweet/and so cold."*
>
> *-William Carlos William*

This chapter's prescription is a two-parter. It is both a food prescription (AKA recipe) that reminds us that no one does it better than Mama Gaia, and it is also a prescription for deepening our presence during meals. A reminder that the "how" of our eating is just as important as the "what" of our eating.

* Of note, please have the following meal for breakfast or later on in the day if you prefer, but always on an empty stomach.

A few RIPE pieces of a fruit of the current season, one that you enjoy (example pears in the fall, tangerines in the winter, and plums in the summer)
A bowl
A beautiful tranquil spot
(optional) eating utensil

Place your ripe fruit in the bowl, settle into your tranquil spot. Give thanks in whatever way that resonates with you for what you about to eat. Begin to eat. Take your time with each piece of fruit, paying attention to fragrance, texture, consistency, and the subtlety of flavors. Close your eyes if you need to, to truly focus on these different aspects of the food. Think of a sommelier tasting wine. Chew well and thoroughly. Also pay attention to the subtle (and sometimes not so subtle) differences in taste from one piece of fruit to the next. Stop eating when sated.

The above experience can be done with someone else and I even recommend it (after having done it on your own a few times). I suggest that when you share in the experience, you either eat *silently* together OR keep the conversation focused on the food and the sensory experience of it. In Joy.

Dance link: Delicious Healing

https://www.youtube.com/watch?v=YVwHVDlvArY

CHAPTER 2

Your Movement practice

Scorpio Cat Woman

I scratched the back of his neck.
That marked the beginning
of the end. Seven months later
in another season entirely, a scorpion
pierced my left heel. I could not breathe
for the pain. I vomited for two days—
spit up mango bits and my old
weaknesses. Walked jagged lines
for a week, aimed for my mouth,
and struck my nose. My blood spilt
with the descent of rain. And in the downfall,
I shed my shame, that old comfortable skin,
and pulled on black boots.

I stretched out.

I scratch now with fewer apologies,
talk hardly ever, but sing more than I
sting. My super powers include
night time vision and clicking my heels
in dance, especially during the eye of
a storm.

-Tumi Johnson

Dr. Tumi Johnson, M.D.

I've decided we are all super heroes. And I don't mean in the way of being able to go through dark periods of life, of being disease survivors and making it through abuse or neglect or poverty. I mean that we are verified super heroes regardless of circumstance, with cerebral as well as physical potential that most of us haven't even begun to tap into. And this is one of the gifts of exercise. It provides us a field in which to investigate this idea and see the truth of it in very measurable ways. It is a benefit of exercise that I think is just one of the many—the experience of and the sharing of our amazing potentials. Exercise is also one of those very few things that if we could, most of us doctors would put in a pill and prescribe to everyone. It's that effective and that much of a "panacea." I can't think of one organ system or dis-ease that some kind of exercise doesn't improve. I think the reason for that is the same as the one why many of us are drawn to sports. And that reason is that exercise/movement/sport is what our bodies were designed to do. And when we don't do enough of it, our bodies don't do so well.

I used to think I didn't like watching sports because while growing up, I was often bored while my dad passionately yelled at the TV, engrossed with NBA basketball and Wimbledon tennis games. But the truth was my attention was just as rapt as his during the Olympics when watching the track and field races, ice skating, and gymnastics. Which leads me to this. All of us are drawn to movement— it may just not be the "popular" movement. I've worked with many people who tell me "Doc, I'm just not into exercise" because their version of exercise is limited to running or bicycling. What about rebounding? What about rollerskating in the park, climbing, cartwheels? My sweetheart loves go karting and the physical and mental stamina he has to generate for this activity, is impressive. What about dancing?? All of this and much much more are all of what I would call exercise. So I dance a little jig inside and restrain myself from doing it on the outside when a patient or client says to me "I'm just not into exercise." Oh yes, you are. You just haven't found *your* movement play. And what, you might ask, is "movement play?" It is the concept and idea I'd like to offer as an alternative to "exercise." I don't exercise, I play.

I first heard this idea while attending the first Woodstock Fruit Festival in New York state in 2011 from Dr. Douglas Graham. A lifetime athlete and advisor to world-class athletes and trainers around the globe, Dr. Graham has worked professionally with top performers in several sports including tennis legend Martina Navratilova, NBA pro basketball player Ronnie Grandson and pro women's soccer player Callie Withers, among others. Doug is also in his sixties and I watched him "play" his way into conquering the field in fitness exercises. A field that was mostly inhabited by twenty something year old very buff looking men. He demonstrated that play is not some physically delayed half-brother to "exercise." Play is actually where it's at. "Play" rather than "exercise" captures the delight aspect of movement that I think is so vital to having an effective and enjoyable fitness practice. I've expanded the term of play to "movement play" because I think there are forms of play that are not physically challenging for the body— an example is a great game of poker or the hand slapping song games I loved playing with my sisters and friends as a girl in Ibadan, Nigeria. *Movement* play, however, IS physically challenging and it is also fun and we've been doing it from our very start. I love hearing from expectant mothers how they can feel their babies doing "cartwheels" and "leaps" and "dancing" in their wombs. We are playing from the time we begin to form our limbs within our mothers' uteri, and those limbs are designed for movement. In fact our entire organism is, and studies show that our lack of movement (for example prolonged sitting) results in a shortened life span[1]. However, what has happened to the majority of us (especially those of us in urban and suburban "civilized" settings), is a steady decline in movement play over the past decades. The amount of children who now are spending much more time on video games (another great example of play that is not movement play) rather than playing outdoors in movement, has reached startling numbers. So are the numbers of schools, especially under-funded ones, who do not have a physical education program for growing children. There are now children who are literally indoors in a classroom for a full day without moving their bodies in play. In this category, I also think about women who are usually of an older generation in the U.S. and multigenerational in many parts of the world. These women attended primary school and secondary school and while there might have been P.E. in their schools, it was seen as a boy's activity and it was not part of the curriculum for the girls. They were offered home economics instead. The lessons of home economics are amazing and I wish I, as my mom had (who outside of her PhD, can efficiently sew beautiful dresses), had received some of those lessons. But not at the expense of having had the opportunity to be on the girls' soccer team in high school. To be a member of a sports team gave me a chance to be a part of a group of teenage girls who at least for 90 minutes during practice or a game, were celebrated for more than our looks but rather our physical skills, tenacity, and teamwork.

And then there are those who *do* have a physical education program in their school and are privy to it, but don't feel lucky about it at all, because as many know who've ever participated in "school group sports," the school playground or sports field can be one in which dramas of peer pressure, popularity contests, and feelings of inadequacy are played out. Many people feel scarred from such experiences and undergo an adverse reaction to words such as "sports" or "exercise." This has nothing to do with one's predisposition for movement (again we are all designed to move and to move well). Instead, it has more to do with the emotional and mental constructs that have been put on something that is so instinctual and a crucial and potentially joyful element of being alive. There is another reason for feeling discomfort around movement play, apart from not being exposed to it while growing up or having trauma around it. And this reason involves people who come from a culture in which physical education was not part of the curriculum. Depending on their lifestyle, some people in this category might be very fit from doing functional movement activities that might be tied to labor — example farming work, transport of items, walking or bicycling regularly as a mode of transport. These are the people I encounter during visits to many rural areas of the "non-developed" world and they are some of the fittest people I've ever met. However, an increasing number of us are moving to urban areas and as more and more areas are getting "developed" and more conveniences are offered, sedentary practices can often take over. Without a practice of movement play, this can can prove detrimental to one's health.

The other aspect of exercise that can feel like a turn-off for some people (though a turn-on for others) is the element of competition. It might be at dance class, a volleyball game, running in the park only to be overtaken by another runner, or at the gym side-eyeing the guy next door lifting more weights than you are. Whatever the setting, feelings such as envy, inadequacy, and unworthiness can come up during sports. It is a paradigm that offers the idea that if the fellow standing next to you can beat your personal best in running, bicycling, insert sport here, he is probably better at everything else in life. It is a paradigm that is often supported by commercial ads and some media, and frankly it's one that is pretty tired. It is one that does not nurture a self-loving or positive mindset. Nor is it the most effective mindset. If you are a runner and you are constantly looking back or sideways at your "competition," you are apt to not run as fast as you can. And even if you "win," you weren't truly present during the "race" because your eye was on others rather than on your path. Some of the best athletes past and present share the same advice when it comes to performing one's best and it can be roughly translated to "compete with yourself, not others." Work on being better than your last time, rather than someone else's. Because that way, when you become the "best" in the field, you keep on improving. With such a philosophy, you see others doing what you do as sources of inspiration to help improve your game, rather than "competition." I can share with you that as a dancer, having that epiphany about dancing (which can be one of the most competitive "sports" out there), resulted in huge leaps—pun intended— in my dancing, and my continued enjoyment of dance. I walked into a dance class and stopped looking at other dancers as my competition for an audition. Rather, I began watching their movements with appreciation and as sources of teachable moments (no matter how they were dancing). I then implemented those lessons in my own dancing, focusing on being better than I had been the day before, rather than comparing my dancing to another. Doing this practice changed my entire experience of dancing for the better.

I hope that's helpful for you to think about re: competition. Just focus on your path with self-kindness no matter what anyone else is doing.

So you may be thinking, "well I don't fit into any of these categories. I'm really into exercise and I do it pretty regularly!" That's fantastic. But here is the question. Are you into exercise the way you're into getting your teeth cleaned? You don't enjoy it but you do it solely because you're afraid of not having a great smile, or even losing those teeth. In other words, you are "into exercise" for fear-based reasons (example: looking too skinny without enough muscle definition, or getting fat, or developing diabetes), but you don't *really* enjoy it. Now I'll be clear. I engage in movement play because I like to look good but also because I truly enjoy it. And this is the key….it gets back to the play and pleasure of it. I've heard many people tell me that they do feel good but only after their "workout" is done. I don't much like that word, by the way, and I'm happy to say I haven't "worked out" in years. What I have done is engaged in movement play and played myself to the strongest, most supple, and fittest body that I've ever had. There are two terms here that are key. The first is "engaged" and the second is "movement play." When people tell me that they've come to expect their "exercise"/"workout" to be a total torture session but then to feel good afterwords, I grow a little concerned. It's true that it can be at times a challenge to get motivated to start one's movement play and that during the session there might be periods of great discomfort. Lacing one's shoes up to go for a run, putting on your clothes and entering the dance studio, strapping on your helmet for the bike ride might all be done with a bit of reluctance some days. However, within a few moments, if you're engaged in a movement practice that you enjoy, that lack of motivation is obliterated by pure joy, even when the practice is very intense physically. Many people don't "engage" in their movement practice for the simple reason that they don't really enjoy it. Think of how many times people are plugged into screens while on the treadmill or stationary bike. I've been told by patients and clients who do this that "it makes the time go faster" which just adds credence to my belief that they need to find a different movement practice. It's the opposite of "engaging" in movement if one is multi-tasking during movement practice; it is actually disengagement and there are few concerns I have with it. One, it's one of the easiest ways to get injured. If you aren't paying attention to the way you're moving, you are likely to get hurt whether in a dramatic slip/fall scenario or a more common insidious injury that comes with not paying attention to your body during exercise. Another concern is that when you "multitask" during your movement practice, you are not present. And apart from the injury risk that comes from not being present, as already discussed, you rob yourself of all the wonderful gifts of presence. These include a sense of calmness, a state of centeredness, honed focus and now-ness in which mind chatter, worry, and thoughts do not penetrate. It's an amazing state to be in and being still in the lotus position is not the the only way to achieve it. Conscious, present movement play can do this. And with it come the enkaphelins and endorphins, the natural "high" that those who are truly in the "zone" of movement, talk about. And that "high" is heightened even more when you love the movement you are doing. Which gets me to the second key term—"movement play." As I mentioned before, joy is really at the center of this concept. Do you enjoy the movement you are doing? Personally speaking, I love to dance and run and do yoga and swim— and by swimming, I don't mean laps, I mean more like frolicking in the water and pretending I'm a mermaid. These movement practices make me happy. And I love trail biking but if you tell me we are going road biking, you've destroyed my high. Biking on the shoulder of paved roads, often in close to proximity to speeding vehicles doesn't do it for me. Sorry. I offer myself as an example simply to show that one movement practice is not right or wrong. Just find one and the kind of one (frolicking mermaid verses butterfly strokes, for example) that works for you. You might prefer group activities or prefer solo. You might prefer activities with lots of "props" or ones that are more minimalist. Ones that incorporate the element of water (like swimming or surfing) or ones that are more about the element of air like acro-yoga, aerial dance, gymnastics. There are also those that incorporate a mixture of the elements: running and dancing (which for me also have elements of both earth and air, and perhaps more of one depending on the type of dancing). You might love movement play that is more creative and interpretive or prefer more structured activity. I think you get my point. There is so much to choose from. And if you are confused, look to the children, which we should do more often. Look to children for ideas that we may have lost (we definitely had them before—remember, movement is our birthright). Look to them more for the pure joy that crosses their faces when they're engaged in movement play that they love. And it's this feeling more than any other that I would use as guidance in choosing your regular movement practice(s). What brings you joy? What movement makes the time fly by? What movement practice helps keep you present to the now so that intrusive thoughts have a harder time making their way in? Do that.

Now, there might be some resistance to this because of the fear that you wouldn't get a balanced exercise regimen doing this. Maybe for example, you feel drawn to yoga as your joyful movement play and you worry that you wouldn't get strong enough or get enough aerobic exercise from this movement form. I've heard this a lot. And any yogi can tell you (or anyone who's gone through a good 90 minute vinyasa, ashtanga, or Bikram class) that you have nothing to worry about. It's my experience that most healthy people, when they allow themselves to do so, intuitively choose joyful movement practices that all together, give them this "balanced exercise regimen," one that strengthens, tones, increases suppleness and provides aerobic fitness. Also, there is one thing that I think is sorely missing in many discussions on exercise. And that is what one is doing when one *isn't* "exercising." Unless you're a professional athlete/mover, you are likely spending much less of your time in scheduled exercise than not. After those 30-90 minutes of working out, what are you doing with the other approximately fifteen hours of your waking life, movement wise? It's not unusual to see this in most cities—someone coming to the gym and taking the elevator up and down before and after one's workout. And that to me is a reflection of the disconnect around movement. I would invite you to consider engaging in movement playing *all day*. It doesn't have to be the fantastic, heart pumping "sweat fest" of your joyful movement play practice, but make the choice all day to move. That is, when you're not resting, which is also crucial for delicious living, and which is coming up in a future chapter. There is a reason why people in "walkable" cities are found to be healthier (although not necessarily happier) than those in non walkable areas[2] and it's been traced to this "non-scheduled" daily exercise. Are you biking and walking and running when you can, rather than choosing more sedentary forms of transportation? And even if you don't live in a "walkable city," there are more choices than one realizes. Do you circle a building block in your car for ten minutes rather than parking ten minutes away and using that same amount of time to walk (when you can walk, don't have too much to carry, and the weather is not abysmal?) Do you take the elevator or escalator that is right next to a staircase when you are able-bodied? Or carry your bags of groceries rather than using a cart when you have just two or three bags to carry? Those are just a few examples of choices. Make it a game of sorts. How can I move more in small ways during the day? Remember play? That's play.

Now. There are some of you who might be thinking "Ah, no. That's going to mess up my look, my hair. I will sweat." Or "I can't do that in my fabulous heels." Well, I am a bonifide dress/skirts kind of woman and I move all the time. Even when I was little, my preferred outfit for biking and skateboarding was a dress. Your personal style does not have to be sacrificed in the name of fitness. Your hair will not get ruined by small sprints up the stairs during the day or walking a few extra blocks to your car, and if it does, you may want to reconsider your hairstyle. Also, in general, if you sweat uncomfortably after the amount of exercise I'm talking about here, trust that as you get more fit, the sweating quantity will decrease. And if it's the smell of your sweat that makes you uncomfortable, then please refer to Chapter 1 on how to improve your diet so that your body no longer emits such an unpleasant odor when you sweat. I will also add this piece of advice as a lover and owner of fabulous heels myself: keep the heels for a special and short-lasting occasion (or bring the comfy shoes to switch out to). However for daily life, find some comfortable shoes that allow you to move freely and when need be, quickly. I happen to think, for example, that huaraches are great, sexy on both men and women, and go with almost everything. In the winter, one can find some stylish and comfortable boots. And if you're a sneakers guy or girl, well you're set. But please move. If vanity is your key concern around this moving all day thing (and that is absolutely fine), I can attest that you will look better very quickly as your body becomes more agile and graceful in daily life with this movement practice. And no outfit can give you that, or the level of confidence that comes with feeling better in your body.

Movement is not just about large actions of the limbs, but also about alignment and posture. How do you move your head in relationship to your spine? Does your head jut out towards your computer or do you spend a lot of the day with your neck flexed looking downward at your mobile device? Many physicians, including myself, are seeing an increase in neck pain and there are studies that show this as well as a connection between increased computer use and neck pain[3,4]. I believe this is in part related to our lack of consciousness around how we move and hold our heads. And your lower spine? When you stand, you are still moving, muscles are firing and you are either lifting (more movement) your spine gently upwards or you are not. You are either moving/keeping your weight evenly on both of your feet soles or you are not. These subtle postural movements take up far more of our time than the usual 30-90 minutes we allot to exercise and yet we don't look at them enough. What I am getting at is the importance of "functional" or every day movement and posture. Some of the healthiest people don't have an "exercise regimen" but they walk regularly, garden, bicycle to work, plant trees, clean their homes, *build* their homes, and they stand or move while working. The last point, "standing or moving while working" is one I'd like to spend a bit of time on since many of us spend six or more hours engaged in our work, and for too many of us, that means prolonged siting. And this sitting is outside of the time we spend sitting at home relaxing to a movie or a TV show, or having a meal. This is detrimental to our health; we are not meant to be sitting for such long periods of time, and studies have shown that there is a link between the amount of time spent sitting and dying prematurely[5]. But if that's not enough to jolt you physically out of your chair, consider that for however long you *do* live, the quality of your life is deeply compromised by prolonged sitting. Back pain, neck pain, which are two of the leading complaints I and other primary care health care providers encounter in the clinic, is often caused and/or worsened by prolonged sitting. Yet, it can be improved dramatically when ergonomic changes are made to one's work environment. As a dancer and doctor, I spend many hours of the day in movement but in the past, I found that I was also spending too many hours of the day sitting, whether in the clinic typing up patient health plans, studying medicine, or doing administrative paperwork. And it was beginning to affect my dancing— I felt more stiff and felt like my core muscles were losing strength. Creating and regular using a standing work desk is one of the most transformational things I did in terms of my fitness. Now, when I am in a session with a client/patient, when I am doing said paperwork, emailing, as I write even this, I am standing. I have a set up in which I have a tall standing desk in front of me and I place my computer on that, ensuring that the screen is on the same "latitude" as my head. This is so that my head is not jutting forwards or bending down as I type. I also ensure that my hands can rest comfortably on the keyboard. More and more work places have moving and standing tables in which you can place your working laptop. And if your work place doesn't have this and you do a significant amount of computer work, I suggest that you inquire about it to your employer(s), saying that you need it for health reasons. Because you do. We all do. More and more organizations are offering more ergonomically flexible work set-ups for their employees because they are aware of the research that healthier (and happier) employees translates to less sick days and greater productivity. It's just smarter business. If you work from home, then I suggest you either buy or create your own standing desk. You do not have to buy an expensive apparatus to achieve this setup (though you can if you prefer). My sweetheart and I travel a lot for both work and pleasure and so we are constantly creating our own standing desks. It's often a fun exercise using the different furniture and other random pieces in our travel spot to create the perfect standing work stations for ourselves. I have included in the references[6] a link to the website my partner created; the website offers some of the creative examples of DIY standing workstations he made during our travels. I cannot speak highly enough of standing and moving while working. Apart from instantly improved posture (if you have the correct setup), key muscle groups like your erector spinae and core muscles as well as well as quadriceps and hamstrings are engaged in a way that is not afforded to them when you are sitting. With your shoulders back in a good position (as opposed to slumped forwards), you breathe better and deeper and there is a relaxed alertness that comes with that. Also, it is my experience that it is hard to stand still for several hours at a time (much harder than sitting) and that is a good thing. Too few of us are taking breaks when we work. Standing while working is a physical reminder for that rest because after about an hour at my standing desk, my body needs a break. I usually take this break by spending 5-10 minutes doing a simple inversion exercise, doing some light stretching with breath work and getting a drink of water before then returning refreshed to my work. Those 5-10 minutes are not a long time but many of us don't give ourselves that rest and instead, sit zombie-like sitting with a worsening slouch and tension, trying to get the work done. We do this for hours daily and believe that the 1hr of gym time a few days a week will erase the harmful effects of this practice. It can't. It can help but why get in that harmed state in the first place? Why not create, as much as you can, a work environment that supports your health rather than detracts from it, especially since many of us spend so much time at work. I love having a standing desk and can't imagine going back to a chair for work. While standing and working, I don't stay entirely still for that hour of work and this I think is helpful for preventing or worsening lower extremity swelling (diet is also key— please again refer to Chapter 1). As I work, I punctuate the static standing by doing heel lifts or doing a few hip and head circles from time to time. I might shift back and forth from foot sole to foot sole. I might do a couple of deep squats. Just a few seconds of this while I work. It instantly returns me to full body consciousness, centers me, and I find that I am re-connected to my breath which can often be lost when we get sucked into a work activity.

I know I have spent a lot of time on this topic but I think it's well warranted and for all the exercise recommendations made out there, this one is not spoken or written about enough. Please take the time to ask yourself how many hours a day you spend sitting. If it's more than three hours (this includes "relaxation time," I strongly urge you to start standing and walking more by using a standing desk for your work and even for some of your home tasks.

"Functional" activities such as gardening/planting trees, "home-work" (vigorous cleaning and upkeep of your home), bicycling to work and walking in your neighborhood may not seem like a feasible lifestyle choice for you, depending on where you live and the nature of your work. However, you can still incorporate some of the above activities no matter where you live, if you are able bodied. Speaking of which, there is a saying in medicine that "the less you move, the less you move." In other words, the more sedentary a person gets, the more the wheels are put in motion for lack of fitness, possible injury, dis-ease and thus, less and less ability to move with ease. The opposite is also the case and one I prefer to say, being a "glass half full" kind of person. "The more you move, the more you move." If you know that your fitness level could improve and you aren't moving enough, it doesn't matter where you are on the "able bodied" scale. Engaging more in movement play will make a positive impact, and result in more and more ease in movement which in turn, results in moving more, and being healthier.

There's another element of movement play that I think is often overlooked and that is *where* we do our movement play. I think it is vitally important as much as we can to engage in play in Nature. Apart from the air provided by oxygen-emitting trees, the visually stimulating and soul elevating beauty that Nature gives us, Nature is also the ultimate "training field." I used to spend a lot of time running on treadmills in gyms— I could really track my pace as well as how long I was going, thanks to all the numbers on the machine. But it's a machine. It's absolutely predictable and it can also be absolutely boring. Nature, on the other hand, gives you slopes and rocks and twists and turns— that no treadmill program can replicate— and so your cognition, your cerebellum which helps with balance, as well as your limbs are all getting a "work out." One of the best ways to increase fitness is the element of surprise, of variety, so that your muscles don't get bored, and are consistently challenged, and that is just what Nature's courses provide. It is yet another example of how "play" is just the smarter option compared to prescribed or rigid "workouts," apart from it being way more fun. There is also a more nuanced benefit of moving in Nature. Nature is our original home, before modernization and districts and high-rises, we were intimate with and co-evolved with Nature's microbiome. It is a part of us in a very real sense and I think this is one reason why so many people feel a sense of calm and familiarity when they are in Nature (I have a whole chapter on this coming up). So moving in Nature also gives one that sense of grounded-ness and comfort that the best homes provide. And this helps to increase one's confidence in movement which in turn, all helps us become more fully who we truly are. And *that* is delicious healing.

My Exercise Prescription (three tips):

1. Check in with yourself about your current "exercise" practice. Do you engage in it mindfully? And even more importantly, do you get a deep sense of joy when you engage in it? If so, you have a movement play practice that is great for you. If not, please start exploring. There are fun online exercises that consider your personality and help you make a match. Personally, I recommend thinking about movement practices that you enjoy watching, what "every day" physical activities bring you joy, and what you loved doing when you were a child in terms of movement. Those are a great place to start.

2. Once you've found your current movement play practices of choice, please engage in it/them at least thrice a week and at least twice a week *in Nature*, if that option is available to you.

3. Purchase or create your own standing work station and begin using it frequently, cutting your sitting time to 3-4 hours max a day.

CHAPTER 3

Meditation/ Mindfulness

Air Hunger

The problem with fantasy— one of them—
is that I forget to breathe. I forget that my body craves
the citrus like ballooning of inhale,
exhale's slow cherry release.

What happens when the appetite is misplaced?

I scramble out of this skin, this wise skin,
use my heart for footing, hoist myself
marsupial like, with eyes to match,
onto a shoulder to crouch then catapult
through a careless sinus into savage cerebrum.

And there, I'm swept along thought highways of
what if and if only. And all the while, this body,
this knowing body whispers, "where have you gone?"
waiting for me to join me. For me to feed my hunger for infinite
impossibility with the only possibility of here.

- Tumi Johnson

As a child growing up, the library was one of my happy places. My family and I moved from Ibadan, Nigeria to Nashville, Tennessee when I was around twelve years old. The local public library was one the few spaces I felt I could completely relax and escape from the angst of a tween girl transplanted into a very different culture from the one I had been used to. Long weekend hours were spent going through the aisles and discovering and devouring poetry collections, novels, memoirs…and Iyengar. One day, rifling through the dance section, I wondered a bit too far and stumbled upon a book the cover of which had a picture of a woman in a bright red leotard, with a long braided ponytail, and bent into an interesting shape. I took the book back to my seat in the library and began reading. After it was time to go, I checked the book out and kept reading. I started trying out the shapes on my own body. I renewed this book as often as I was able to until I'd memorized most of the sequences. The book was Yoga: The Iyengar Way by B.K.S. Iyengar, and it was the beginning of my journey into yoga. I read this book and began practicing yoga about six years before yoga really began taking off in America and I think what captivated me was that the thirteen year old burgeoning dancer in me recognized grace, great alignment, strength and presence even at that age, and I wanted some. By this time, I was having asthma attacks still very frequently and I found that the poses that I did, along with the instructions on breathing, helped decrease the frequency of these attacks. And if the attacks *did* begin, in general, they didn't become as severe.

Yoga, and I didn't know it yet, was also wonderful training for dance. Bringing in that element of mindfulness to my movement was something that did and continues to significantly improve the quality of my dancing.

At the heart of yoga, and what I would like to share with you in this chapter, is mindfulness. We may come to a mindfulness practice through many avenues— time spent in nature, a relationship with a pet (animals are incredible teachers of presence), through other mindful movement practices like qi gong, or a sport that requires one's total attention. But the underlying connecting theme is the same—true mindfulness. And it has been my professional and personal experience that a regular intentional practice in mindfulness is a game changer for one's health.

Mindfulness is a bit of a funny word because anytime we experience it, it often comes as the opposite of a "full" or busy mind. What the word really is getting at is awareness, presence. It's not about the absence of thought but rather, a slightly dis-attached observing stance towards those thoughts. This inevitably results in a quieting of the mind. In the next chapter, I will focus on rest and sleep but it was important for me to separate the chapter on that with this one on mindfulness. There is a key difference between the two realms, though I believe both are crucial for optimal well-being. Mindfulness is a state of restful alertness. You can be very much alert while being at peace, and mindfulness offers this, a gift that is an incredible tool as we navigate through life. Sleep, on the other hand, just as important, has to do with a decreased/different state of consciousness and that while restful, is not alert.

There are an increasing amount of studies that demonstrate the benefits of a mindfulness practice on one's health and happiness, helping to heal conditions ranging from depression and PTSD to diabetes, and being overweight[1-4].

Sometimes when I ask, "do you have a meditation practice?" I get a response such as the following: "all life is meditation," or "I just try to LIVE meditation." The first sentence is true and the second, the ultimate goal but very few of us (especially living with the modern life stressors) are "living" meditation without an intentional practice. Even monks secluded from many of these stressors and living in beautiful and remote natural settings, have an intentional practice of meditation. Ironically, those who often give me the above responses seem pretty agitated. Apart from the studies cited above, I have definitely found that having an intentional and consistent practice in mindfulness is profoundly centering. It has provided me with a deep sense of peace even in the face of changing circumstances, and also helped tremendously with me making the best choices for my life. The last point is one I'd like to address because it's one I hadn't read/heard about before starting to meditate and yet I think it is a powerful incentive to start such a practice. When I began setting aside time daily for meditation, coming into a state of deep present awareness, I began to hear something. Growing up in the church, I often heard about "that still small voice" that was a representation of Spirit within. When I started meditating regularly, I finally got it. And it's the best way I can describe what I hear. It is a serene yet sure voice that feels like myself and also beyond myself. And I always know it's that voice and not mind chatter because of the calmness and love infused in it, the expansiveness I feel when hearing it, and because frankly, it's brilliant. Usually when I get the instruction or the advice from my inner voice, I smile because it's so perfect or my eyes fly open with excitement or an eyebrow goes up in surprise. It is that voice that told me to start my holistic medical practice, to dance more, to go to Thailand at a time that didn't make logical sense where I met the most wonderful man I had ever known. It was that voice that told me that this book needed to be written in this way and at this time. Some might call the voice God, others Source, others Spirit, others Self, others Madness. Apart from the last one (it feels like the opposite of madness), I resonate with all of these names. But what I think is more important than the name or label is one's experience and relationship with the voice. I don't always hear instruction; sometimes it is just a feeling of deep peace and sometimes it is simply the awareness of my extreme mind chatter. However, just that awareness alone can bring me even more into the present.

So perhaps you were piqued reading about some of the health benefits of a meditation practice. Or maybe I had you at "hearing voices," or maybe you're already interested in a meditation practice but have problems starting and/or sticking to one. Whichever category you might be in, your question is probably now, "how?" How does one choose, begin, and stick to a meditation practice?

Yoga was my avenue into a meditation practice because eventually, after all the reading and practice on my own, I found myself in yoga class. During Savasana (corpse) pose which is done usually at the end of class, as a way to "seal" the movement practice, I had a teacher who guided us through a stillness meditation session that lasted just five minutes. However, those five minutes resulted in a feeling of such calm within me and it was enough to motivate me to look more into meditation.

Before this, I was experiencing mindfulness through my challenging yoga asana practice and also through another movement practice I loved— dancing. It was especially during these two activities that my mind would become so focused on the movement and my breath, that nothing else was really filtering in. And this was quite physically and mentally refreshing, and restorative. However, we are not constantly engaged in challenging movements that make it easy to be present due to their demand of our focus. In fact, the majority of the time we are not, and this is when mind chatter can increase and when thoughts wander in and take seats or start rearranging the furniture without us even being aware they have moved in. And this is why I think a stillness and/or "easy movement" meditation practice is key. I define an "easy movement" meditation practice as one that doesn't feel physically or mentally challenging and so the mind can easily wander. This, as well as a stillness meditation practice I think are fantastic for becoming aware of the thoughts that do come in. And awareness is the first vital step for transformation.

An "easy movement" meditation practice for you might be yin yoga or t'ai chi or a simple walking meditation but for others, these very examples might *not* count as "easy movement" meditation because they find the movements physically or mentally challenging and so the mind does not wander at all. Each person is different.

Stillness meditation practices in contrast, for basically everyone, provide the perfect opportunity for increased awareness of thoughts because there is no conscious purposeful movement occurring, and so all focus can be on the experience of observing the mind.

There are stillness meditation practices that are called more "focus" practices— and they use either a word/phrase (mantra) or a physical object/point of focus (dristi) as a means to guide us back to the present when the mind begins to wander. There are also stillness meditation practices that are more "awareness" practices— simply being aware of your mind and using breath or sensation to guide you back to the present. There are also guided meditation practices, in which your mind is led on a journey through words, story, and/ or images, and it is this guiding voice that is meant to help keep you present.

I often have clients and patients who get concerned about which meditation is right or correct. All of it is right and correct. Just do the one that resonates with you at this time. That might change for you in the future but recognize that all of them have basically the same purpose. Whichever one you have available to you, that excites you to try, and that you experience the most benefit from, that's the one for you. Just get started.

Just get started and then stay consistent. The latter is key.

I had a wonderful instructor during my yoga teacher training who shared with us how transformational her Vipassana course had been. Before then, I'd never heard of Vipassana and something in me responded with a sound "yes" to what she was talking about. What she was talking about was a ten day silent meditation course in a retreat center with other people who were in practice just as you, with both group and individual meditation periods, meditating around ten hours a day for ten days straight. During this ten day period, you would also be guided daily, learning how to deepen into self awareness through meditation. As they say, when the student is ready, the teacher will appear. And I was ready. I did my first Vipassana retreat in the Joshua Tree desert in Southern California; it was life changing in so many ways and it greatly strengthened my meditation practice. About a year after my retreat, I was spending time with a friend of mine who had also done Vipassana retreat; however, she had not continued a regular meditation practice after the retreat was over and she was contemplating returning for a second 10 day retreat but was hesitant. When I asked her what was holding her back from returning, she told me that during her first retreat, she met a woman who cheerfully told her that it was her sixth retreat. My friend commented to the woman that (since it was her sixth time around) she must have a very strong home practice! To this, the woman replied that she didn't have a home meditation practice at all and was hoping this sixth retreat would be the trick to help her stick to meditating regularly. I share this story not to dissuade anyone from attending meditation retreats. I think they can be amazing and I have experienced that reality; furthermore, even if one doesn't stick to regular meditation after such a retreat, the sheer practice of taking a retreat is self-caring and healing in of itself. However. Just as one goes for a detox retreat or to a "fitness camp" and then returns home to resume a poor diet or a sedentary lifestyle, it is likely not anyone's goal to go to a meditation retreat only to return home and drop the practice all together.

So while retreat is an amazing first step and can be wonderful to do at intervals (I love to do some sort of meditation retreat yearly), the question is "how does one create a home meditation practice that sticks?"

Dr. Tumi Johnson, M.D.

The short answer is to *do whatever works for you*. The longer answer is here in the form of seven tips— they are just suggestions based on my personal experience and also the experience of working with so many people who when I ask them about their mediation practice, respond by saying, "I used to meditate but then I sort of stopped..."

If you find yourself having a hard time being consistent, here are a few tips that might help:

1) Do it at the same time every day. We are definitely creatures of habit and pairing activities to a certain time of day can help re-enforce the habit (think brushing teeth before bed for example).

2) Speaking of when to do it, as with exercise, I have found it helpful to meditate first thing in the morning, before excuses and unplanned events get in the way.

3) Keep it simple. Just stay in bed to do it if you have to. I know someone who fell out of his meditation practice because he had created a beautiful meditation spot in his home and during the winter he had a hard time motivating himself to get out of bed and go to said spot to meditate. So he stopped meditating altogether. Keep it simple.

4) Use apps. There are increasing numbers of them. I use one on my phone called Insight Timer that I'm pretty happy with (I do not get any sponsorship or kickbacks from them, I'm simply sharing my experience). It has a few meditation bells that I like and it also has a feature that lets you know how many people are meditating with you at the same time that you are. It's a lovely feature that underscores our connectedness, and can be motivating. This feature, along with the optional feature of "friending" people on the app which allows you to see when they meditated last, was really helpful to my mother for staying consistent. She sent me a friend request and loves seeing when I meditate. There was

a moment when I completed meditation and a message came up on the app that my mother who was across the world at the time, had also just finished meditation. It was a wonderful moment. This feature might sound like your worst nightmare and even stalker-ish— again it's optional— but my point is there are some great apps out there as simple or as complex and individualized as you like, and they can truly help support your practice.

5) Recognize that even just ten or twenty minutes of regular meditation will make a positive difference (just like exercise). Again, the key is consistency.

6) Especially if time is a challenge for you, it's helpful to know and remind yourself that doing this practice allows for greater efficiency with your work and sharper focus with all your activities. So here's a great mind hack: if you're short on time, you can't afford *not* to meditate!

7) Release expectation. You might think after starting your meditation practice "Where is the voice???" "I can't hear the @#&$# 'still voice'!" Please release expectation around hearing guidance. Also, and this is an even more common expectation about meditation, release the one on having 'a blank mind' that is serenely free of any thought. I had one patient who said to me once, "I failed at meditation. I just couldn't stop my thoughts." I believe that you can't "fail" at meditation. Simply the act of becoming still with the intention to quiet one's mind and deepen in awareness IS meditation. The thoughts might come, they usually do. After some meditation sittings, I am simply more aware of my thoughts, but that is also a significant benefit of meditation and an important step in becoming free from those thoughts.

8) The last tip I would offer here for staying consistent with your practice might seem contradictory to the earlier story I shared, and it is to attend one or more meditation retreats.

I can compare this to one's diet, in terms of having both a seasonal cleanse/detox as well as one's maintenance diet. What you are doing most days of the year in terms of what you are eating is more vital than the 7 to 14 days on average one engages in a detox twice a year or so; however, those 7 to 14 days can be amazing in re-enforcing one's healthy eating practices and up-leveling one's diet. Similarly, while I think one's daily meditation practice is what is paramount to consider, a yearly or seasonal meditation retreat can be wonderful in deepening and strengthening one's practice. And it is doesn't have to be away from home. For a few years now, I have created a meditation retreat right in my own home. I simply clear out the schedule for 1-3 days, turn off and put away my computer, turn my phone off, and prepare sustenance ahead of time for those decided days of retreat. This is usually green juices and fruit as I have also found that for me, a nutritional cleanse is perfect during a meditation retreat. I then spend this time "in retreat." For others, the idea of staying home for retreat might be stressful and a break from the familiar might be desired; in that case, leave. There are a plethora of meditation retreat centers around the globe. And separate from meditation centers, depending on your goals and what resonates with you, there are other places that might be even better suited sites for retreat. This might look like a detox/spa center which provides bodywork treatments in addition to a sanctuary of space for you to meditate. Or it might be a yoga retreat center that combines asana/flow practice with breath work and meditation. Or maybe (one of my favorites), you just retreat into Nature with no schedule but that of Nature's rhythms and whims, and no center but the the center within you, and no company but (and take your pick), a waterfall, a stream, trees, the big wide ocean.

I hope you find one, some, or all of the above tips useful in supporting you to establish a consistent meditation practice because again, like with a maintenance diet, it truly can be so sustaining for one's mental and emotional sense of centeredness and peace. This has definitely been the case for me.

That said, I would like to revisit one of the common replies I mentioned to the question I sometimes pose of "do you meditate?" Remember the answer "my LIFE is meditation" (or something akin to that)? That answer used to result in me quelling a roll of the eyes with a bit of disbelief and a tinge of envy. Because it's true, life does offer a continual practice of true presence. However, again, very very few of us are able to achieve this state of mindfulness and staying in the now, constantly. That said, I think it's a wonderful thing to work towards; a daily meditation sitting practice as above helps tremendously with this, but I think something else is often needed. I witnessed this in my own life. After starting a daily meditation practice, I felt an overall sense of deeper calm and centeredness; however, especially on stressful days, I would end the day feeling still quite depleted or I would have an interaction and find myself reacting in a very different way than the self that had emerged from sitting meditation that very morning. So I started having "re-centering breaks" and they have been wonderful both for myself (the guinea pig) and those patients and clients in need of this kind of intervention, to whom I teach this practice.

"Re-centering breaks," as I call them, are carved out moments of time, usually as brief as 1 minute but often about 3-10 minutes, during which I take a pause in my day to intentionally practice mindfulness and by doing so, feel more re-centered and embodied. These breaks can consist of whatever mindfulness practice you enjoy; I personally use a combination of breath work and stretching for my re-centering breaks but again, do whatever resonates with you and that is most effective for quickly bringing you back into the present and into a more balanced state. I suggest that the activity you do during the breaks be something that you feel comfortable doing in most places, including public places (unless you spend virtually the entire day alone and at home). This is one of the reasons I find breath work as a wonderful re-centering break practice: you can do it anywhere, in a meeting, on a crowded subway, in crosstown traffic and no one except you, is the wiser. One simple breath practice that I learned from Dr. Andrew Weil's work is the cycle of inhaling for four counts, holding the breath for seven and exhaling for eight counts. Doing this cycle 3 times is very effective for relaxation and increased presence[5]. Other activities that are great for re-centering other than breath work and stretching include (but are not limited to) journaling, grounding in nature via standing and walking barefoot on the earth or sun gazing, and an inversion exercise. An inversion exercise can be a simple forward bend folding over at the waist if standing and letting your head relax and drop towards your feet. Other great inversions include lying on one's back and lifting one's legs to rest them against a wall, or else a headstand, shoulder stand, or handstand. These are amazingly effective especially when coupled with breathing for feeling both relaxed and extremely energized, and for bringing one firmly into the now. I also encourage scheduling one's re-centering breaks not in a rigid way as in specific hours of the day but rather, more in the way people schedule their teeth brushing (right after waking up or after your breakfast etc). In the same way, you can schedule your re-centering breaks for example, before your mid-morning snack or a water-break, before lunch, in the afternoon right after your workday is done, or after every 1-2 hours of work. Choose whenever works for you, but I recommend doing it not once but a few times a day, especially if you find yourself feeling more tense, anxious, and/or drained than you'd like at the end of the day. Breaking up the day with these above pauses help to reinforce the benefits of your daily meditation practice.

The final thing I want to mention about all of this— re-centering breaks and a daily meditation sitting session and perhaps seasonal or yearly meditation retreats, has to do with time. I have had many clients and patients say to me after I recommend some of the above, "there is just no way. I just don't have the time for this." And frankly, after experiencing the time saving effects of mediation I would counter, "you don't have the time *not* to do this." If you are feeling time-starved, ADDING in more meditation is one of the most effective things you can do. How does this math work? I have found that by taking multiple re-centering daily breaks, I effectively "stop" before starting my next task of the day. That, combined with my daily meditation sitting, keeps me in a state of "flow" and synchronicity and all I can tell you, is that ideas come quicker and easier, conversations and interactions are more harmonious and work tasks unfold more efficiently. I am not alone in this. I think anyone who has daily mindfulness practices can attest to the above. SN Goenka, whose work I learned about during my study of Vipassana, encouraged people to meditate 2 hours every day, reassuring the inevitable fear around lost time by speaking on just the above: work and life unfolds with more flow. If this seems like juju or nonsense, then I encourage you to put it to the test for one month. And then witness "magic" occur. If I were to get scientific about what happens with the above, I would say simplistically the following. Each time you practice embodiment and hone your practice of presence (as the above exercises do), through breath work you improve circulation to your brain, which leads to better, smarter choices throughout the day. And on a more nuanced level, any time you do these exercises, you are taking time for yourself in an intentional self-loving act. And that, I think is one of the most powerful things one can do for having a healthy and happy life.

My Prescription for taking a Re-centering Break:

1. Choose an activity that you feel comfortable doing anywhere at any time and that quickly "drops" you back into your body and into the present. Some possibilities include a breathing sequence, stretching, a mindful movement sequence (yoga, t'ai chi, qu'i gong, or just a few mindful neck stretches and shoulder circles).
2. Decide WHEN in the day you would like to do this activity to help with re-centering. Choose a minimum of twice during the day. I recommend doing it during especially higher stress and/or monotonous periods of the day (as part of your work breaks, for example).
3. Schedule it in, just as you would a meeting. Put it on your daily schedule/calendar, scheduling at least 5 minutes for this break.
4. Engage in this activity every day for at least one week.
5. Check in with yourself about how you feel after the week. Tweak the activity or the timing as needed. And start again. *Start again.*

CHAPTER 4

Sleep and Rest

The Rooftop

Sometimes in all the movement, I am stung
by a calling to stillness. Above the fray,
elevated over the tides of constant motion.
Where is your rest point?

Oh how I love a good rooftop.

Here I have an alertness, a calm, closer to the tips
of mountains, the breeze off a hawk's wing, the tails
of clouds. My eyes clear.
And from this vista, there is a
dawning that
all is unknown, and it is with trust
that I slowly ripple down into the marketplace of the living
but now in my own rhythms, with the language of all
that is elevated.

- Tumi Johnson

In University, to make ends meet, I worked part time as a coffeehouse
barista and often worked the first shift, opening up the coffeeshop in
the early morning hours. I remember even to this day the group of
bleary-eyed students waiting for their first cup of coffee like people
line up at the pharmacy to fill their prescriptions. And often, one
or more of them would tell me (or each other) about the deficit of
sleep he or she had built up. One would say how this was his second

all-nighter in the week. Another would counter how he had been up for 96 hours straight. The interesting thing in all this was always the tone of pride in their voices. And let's be clear. They did not look great. They looked like they were depleted and in need of way more sustenance that a double espresso could provide. And I was no better. I attempted my first all-nighter of my life in University, staying up with the guy I was seeing at the time, to try and finish some paper. I can't even remember the paper. I do remember that I felt like a failure because by 3 am, my brain felt foggy and by 4:30am, I was uncontrollably nodding into sleep and then jerking myself up looking at the clock and hoping the night would be done soon. And the terrible effects of sleep deprivation lasted for a couple of days since, due to a full day's schedule of classes, I wasn't able to catch up on sleep. I could feel it in dance class and rehearsals as decreased physical endurance, in my increased level of irritability with my friends, and in the cloudy judgment around seemingly small decisions. My body and mind were just not the same.

I attempted no more all-nighters in University and surprisingly in Medical school as well, though that is not to say that I was rested— I was often sleep deprived. But during my three years of medical residency, the sleep deprivation climbed to a whole new level and I don't joke when I say that I think it took me more than an entire year after residency was over, to recover both physically and mentally from those years of lack of rest.

And there is no bragging about this. Not anymore at least. Because my recovery just wasn't on the physical level. During my health and personal growth journey, one of the hard realizations about how I as a doctor was sabotaging my own health, was that I had begun to link my identity with sleep deprivation, specifically sleep deprivation that is tied to work. Insidiously, I had somehow bought into the idea that having a 'good work ethic' meant sacrificing sleep more than occasionally. Burning one's candle at both ends, so to speak, in the name of work, especially work that is meant to be of service to others, was something that I had started to think of as a badge of honor. It was in short, the "martyr complex" and for true saints, maybe it works. For me, and for many other doctors that I knew, it was not working. For those who operate under this idea that sleep and rest deprivation is commendable and is a reflection of you being a good care provider (whether healer, parent, etc), I will say the following. What I witnessed and experienced were different levels of resentment that started brewing around feeling physically, mentally, and emotionally run down for the "sake of others." Work ethic does not have to equate to suffering and the masochistic practice of recurrent sleep deprivation, and calling this a good work ethic, even as one's health and/or relationships begin to deteriorate, is a disservice to ourselves, to those we are trying to serve, and to the good work we want to create.

If this writing about work ethic and feeling a sense of pride around self flogging for one's work, resonates with you, or is triggering for you, I invite you to ask yourself the following question:

What does it mean about myself if I spend more time resting and less time working?

If you find that you have judgments around your sense of worth based on how much you work, then please consider doing some inner work around that. I believe that our worth is irrevocable and is not based on how much we work. As a dear old friend of mine once told me, borrowing from Kurt Vonnegut, "you are a great human being, not a great human do-ing."

One of the biggest hurdles around creating more rest for oneself that I observe, is truly believing that you *deserve* more rest. Which is why I have spent so much time on the ego-centric attachment around sleep-deprivation, always doing, lack of rest and being a good person.

Divesting oneself of this illusion is freeing and the first crucial step to creating more rest time for yourself. And one more thing. If you are still stuck with the idea that the more you do in your work (whatever that might be), the more whoever is receiving the benefits of said work, will thrive, I'd like to you to consider this: when we overtax our bodies and minds and don't get the rest we need, irritability, resentment and poorer decision making capabilities inevitably occur. And all those are often felt by the very people we are trying to help. Conversely, sufficient rest gives us energy, supports our best mood which improves both our work and our interactions with those for whom we are working. In addition, loving yourself enough to prioritize rest/self care is a wonderful empowering example of self love to show those around you (whether it be your patients, clients, employees, or children). So please do everyone else a favor, not just yourself, and start prioritizing rest.

I have intensely personal knowledge and experience around the lack of rest. And I witness over and over again, with some of my patients, how the lack of it sabotages all areas of their health, not to mention their happiness. And when I speak about rest, I am not just referring to sleep. In this chapter, I would like to address sleep time rest, waking time rest, and also two other forms of rest that I don't think are discussed enough in this capacity, and that I am excited to share with you.

I hope the above rant has been convincing of your deservedness of rest in all senses of the word.

First, let's begin with sleep time rest and look at the medical literature about the effect lack of sleep has on one's health. There is more and more on this every year. One of the most important ones of recent years is a meta-analysis study reviewing sixteen previous studies that were conducted over 25 years. The researchers of the study found that sleep deprivation was linked to a shorter life span and that those who slept for less than six hours a night on average were 12 percent more likely to experience a premature death[1]. Also, regardless how long your life is, lack of sleep has very real detrimental consequences on the quality of that life. A study coming out of the University of California, San Francisco[2] looked at the relationship between average sleep quantity and getting sick from the common cold. The study's aim was to investigate how poor sleep affects the immune system and it sought to do this by looking at the relationship between sleep and one's susceptibility to the common cold. The study researchers recruited 164 healthy people ranging from ages 18-55 who were then quarantined and infected through nasal drops with rhinovirus (the virus that causes the common cold). Afterwards, the participants were observed for five days to see who actually got symptoms of the cold. The results revealed that those who slept less than six hours a night were four times more likely to have the cold than those who slept more than seven hours a night! Outside of immunity, sleep deprivation is a risk factor for developing type II diabetes[3,4] and has been shown to increase one's risk of overeating and is linked to obesity[5,6]. Sleep deprivation is also strongly associated with depression and anxiety[7,8], increases one's risk of heart disease[9], as well as impairing hormone balance[10], which can compromise fertility. That's the short list. And then there is the very obvious fact that sleep deprivation makes us slower and more forgetful, with poorer reaction and decision capabilities, and that translates to more accidents. In the U.S, the National Highway Traffic Safety Administration estimated that fatigue was the cause in 70, 000 auto crashes and 800 deaths in 2013, though as the Center for Disease Control states, these numbers are likely underestimates[11].

I also think it's important to think not just about how much sleep you are getting but *when* you are getting that sleep. When I returned to New York City from West Africa after my work there as a field doctor for Doctors Without Borders, I began working as a Nocturnalist in a busy well known academic hospital in the city. This meant that I was working strictly night shifts as a doctor in the hospital. Anyone who works graveyard shifts (whether in or out of the home) and tries to get sleep during the day knows the importance of the timing of one's sleep. Daytime sleep is a very poor substitute for nighttime sleep, especially in the long-term. A recent large U.S study found that those who work at least three nights a month are more likely to develop heart problems in the future than those who stick to daytime shifts[12]. Prior studies have also shown links between night time shift work and increased rates of depression, overweight, and possibly increased risk for diabetes[13,14,15]. These medical literature findings are not surprising when one considers that humans have evolved to have a circadian rhythm that is dependent on light and a certain timing of light exposure. There is a disruption of this rhythm that occurs when we are exposed to light during the night. Our eyes which contain light receptors, communicate with the hypothalamus gland (the "mothership" of sorts of our endocrine system) and in turn, this begins a cascade of signals that are channelled through our entire body that has powerful effects on our hormones. These hormones are not just limited to melatonin but also cortisol, serotonin and more, and over time, these continued disruptions can lead to disease, as illustrated by the above studies.

Outside of the physiologic reasons for why it is vital to sleep as much as possible during the night hours, there is another very primal reason, and that has to do with our connection with Nature. Prior to modern conveniences which permitted us to function during the night without the sun's light, as we would in the day, we were basically forced to cease most activity when the sun went down. And there is far more natural wisdom to that than we give credence to.

So that's sleep time rest. But what about the effect of wakeful rest on health? There is a lot of literature on meditation and its positive effects on health, and many could convincingly argue that meditation counts as wakeful rest. That might be true, but in the definition

I would like to put forth in this book, waking rest is different from meditation in two key ways: it is completely unstructured, and there is no one intentional conscious activity being done. So with this definition, knitting, reading, watching television, internet surfing do not count as waking rest. They might feel rest-full to you, although in more cases than you might realize, your body does NOT view these activities as such. This is particularly the case with what I call screen time (internet surfing, video games, watching TV, social media scrolling etc). There are studies showing that there is often a release of dopamine in our brains when we over-engage in these types of screen time activities[16]. And if there is a lot of screen time engagement as there is increasingly for many of us, dopamine receptors begin to become depleted. More than that, the communication pathways (the white matter of our brain) between different vital lobes of our cerebrum become compromised. Actual gray matter might be restructured as well[17]. This is the opposite of rest and it can create dis-ease in the body.

So I don't count screen time engagement as rest. As for knitting, I think it can be seen as a form of meditation when one is in the flow of it. But not wakeful rest in the way I define it above. And reading can provide incredibly valuable information or take us to worlds that are amazingly inventive and creative; but they are someone else's creation. Which leads me to the core reason I don't view any of these activities as waking rest. They don't allow for boredom.

"Wait," you might ask. "Boredom?? Why would I want to go there?" It turns out that carving out and living in a space of unstructured time and doing absolutely *"nothing"* in that time is vitally important for creativity and imagination[18,19]. Boredom is when daydreams can happen. Einstein reportedly said two things about imagination that I love: "Imagination is more important than knowledge" and "Imagination...is the preview of life's coming attractions." Where in our lives do we make time to get "bored," and through that magic of boredom, dream, imagine, and perhaps come up with the next brilliant idea that can positively shift our lives or the lives of our fellow beings? I remember as a girl spending time on a sturdy limb of our backyard grapefruit tree, looking through the overhanging leaves at the clouds, and creating stories in my head. Stories I would later write down as poems. It was lying on my back in the grass where I would often imagine myself dancing on a stage. I would see the movements and then later after daydreaming, I would start to move as I had seen in my head. This was dance class before I knew dance class existed as an option to me. This was my first and probably one of the most important trainings as a dancer. I had this one fantasy that would shift from time to time but it basically looked like gathering all the people around town that looked tired, unwell, or unhappy. I would gather them in our home, prepare and give them some sort of medicinal tonic, offer them a healing bath laced with soothing oils, and create individualized poultices of herbs for each one. They would leave in time, skipping down the street, feeling restored, beautiful, and strong. I had that recurring fantasy when I was little and I think it's really why I became a doctor. Imagination is powerful. But outside of childhood, very few of us are taking time for it. And even within childhood, more and more children in this era of smartphones and video games and over-structured playtime, are missing out on the benefits of "boredom" and waking true rest.

And then there is digestive rest. It can also be called fasting, though in my experience that term seems to strike fear and suspicion in many. Perhaps this is due to religious associations with fasting as well as a common Western societal reading of it as "extreme," unsafe, and tinged with fanatic or cultish undertones.

Fasting, yes, almost always invokes a mental and emotional rest along with a digestive one (they are interconnected). For many, including myself, it also offers a spiritual restoration, but for simplicity sake, in this chapter and in this book, I will be writing about fasting from the digestive rest point of view.

Digestive rest to me is two fold. One aspect of it involves feeding one's body with food that the body recognizes as such (as in whole, natural foods) so that the body can easily process and digest one's meals. Another aspect of digestive rest however, is giving the body enough time away from digestion. And an increasing amount of people around the world are doing this less and less. Many people are "grazing" on significant quantities of several processed meals throughout the day. And the problem with that, among many, is that our bodies never get a break. I have encountered this a lot in clinic when a patient feels unrefreshed after sleep even though she/ he is getting eight hours of sleep routinely a night. Which is reason number 100 for why taking a recent diet history is foundational for me in my medical practice. The processing of food— the digestion and assimilation of nutrients— takes up a significant portion of the body's energy and as it turns out meals with higher protein content require our body to expend more energy than meals with higher content of carbohydrates or fats[21]. As discussed earlier in this chapter, crucial cellular repair and recovery of the body occurs during sleep. This important repair work can thus be compromised if the body is spending time digesting food (especially the more energy requiring high protein meals) or dealing with the inflammation brought on from processed foods.

There are a few simple ways to optimize a restful period away from digestion. I use all three but you can start with whichever one you feel most drawn to. The first is to minimize grazing. Give your body the ability to rest from digesting before then introducing more food to it at the next meal. The second way to give yourself a restorative period away from food is to extend the period of time between your last meal of the day and the first meal of the next day. Eating early in the evening and then not until you are hungry the next day which might not be till past 11 am, is another way to do so. Most people know of and have felt the positive effects of not eating late at night before bed—relief from heartburn and the improved energy and restfulness the morning after, are just two of these effects. However, many people also balk at the idea of not having breakfast early the next morning. When I eat with someone who doesn't know me very well and they find out that this is my first meal of the day and it's noon or 1pm, and that I do this regularly, they often ask "isn't it unhealthy to skip breakfast?" This is fascinating to me because breakfast means literally "to break one's fast" and that can be done at any time of the day. However, people (including me in the past) are socially conditioned to believe that breakfast has to happen by 8 or 9 in the morning unless it's Sunday brunch. Or they read something that convinced them that their metabolism and overall health are compromised if they don't eat early in the morning; that one's metabolism needs a 'jumpstart.' This has not been borne out in sound medical literature. The only two populations that come to mind who are exempt from my above recommendations are elite athletes who are actively training throughout the day and pregnant women. Their nutrient requirements as well as the metabolic and hormonal changes that occur due to their circumstances, may prevent the above schedule.

The third and final way I would offer here for giving your body digestive rest is through a body-directed fast. What I mean by that is that when you feel a lack of appetite (either due to physical or mental or emotional dis-ease, be it as examples, a viral infection or a death of a loved one that takes one's appetite away), honor that by not eating. There has been a lot of misinformation around being physically ill and eating, people believing they need to eat *more* to "fight off" their infection, for example. They hold on to this belief even when their bodies are producing symptoms such as anorexia (a complete lack of appetite or desire to eat), nausea, and abdominal pain. I'll offer a concrete example: acute pancreatitis. Depending on its severity, it results in all the above symptoms. The standard medical treatment includes fasting, made less "woo woo" perhaps by the clinical term "NPO (nothing per oral)." But the same treatment is often recommended for virtually any other *acute* physical dis-ease if your body is giving you signals of temporary lack of appetite. Unless you are suffering from a chronic problem in which your body's signals are skewed (such as major depression, an eating disorder, advanced cancer or a deranged endocrine system with inappropriate hunger/satiety cues), if and when you have no appetite, I invite you to honor that, and fast. That might look like just water and perhaps herbal medicinal teas or as your appetite slowly returns, green juices, or whole natural ripe fruit and vegetables.

The same goes for addressing mental/emotional unrest. For reasons I talked about in Chapter 1 and will talk about more in the following chapter, eating when feeling agitated is a terrible idea on several levels, only one of which is digestion. For those of you who are thinking after reading this, "Well I'm in trouble. Feeling agitated is my state of being most of the time," please check out Chapter 3 and stay there for a while, if you haven't gotten a chance to do so.

There is also a case apart from physical dis-ease or mental/emotional unrest that I think offers another opportunity for body-directed fasting. And that is when we feel "called" to do so. This tends to happen to me when I am traveling across multiple time zones, when I am in a crucial stage of a creative project, and when there is a turn of the season. Basically when a natural but significant shift in my life and/or on the planet is occurring. When this happens, all of a sudden, I feel this natural draw towards fasting. This may not occur for you nor may it be something you resonate with. No problem, as I always say, please do only that which you are drawn to, at this time.

I have written about sleep-time rest, wake time rest, and digestive rest. But this chapter would not be complete without talking about

a type of rest that has been revealing itself to me in recent years—
what I call "New Moon time rest." I am not talking about sleeping
again here, but about the moon cycle of a woman and the amazing
gift that is offered during a woman's new moon time. If you are a
man and your eyes are already glazing over, please stay with me for
a moment. It has been my experience that the rest offered during a
woman's new moon time is not just beneficial for her but for the men
in her life as well. In several communities around the globe in the
past, there was an understanding of the power of the moon and of
women being lunar creatures whose feminine powers, strengthened
and honed through this unique connection with Nature, was a boon
and blessing to the community. It is an understanding that I think
has been widely forgotten as we as a people stepped further and
further away from this connection with Nature (more on this in
Chapter 6). But that connection is there even when we are ignorant
of it. And I think it is the *absence* of honoring this connection as
a woman that can lead to issues as "benign" as having an irregular
or moderately uncomfortable menstrual flow cycle, to as severe as
debilitating pain that disrupts sexual pleasure and daily functioning,
and that even possibly creates tumors in one's womb. This often
comes with the psychic distress of feeling that the very parts that
"make you a woman" are attacking you. I've worked with many
women with these issues including dysmenorrhea, dyspareunia,
uterine fibroids, endometriosis, among other diagnostic names and
quite often, there is a disconnection between the woman and her
moon cycle. One way to heal this disconnection and thus powerfully
heal some of the above issues, is for women who are still experiencing
menstrual flow (i.e. pre-menopausal women), to reconnect with
their cycles. Among other ways of doing this include tracking one's
cycle (being aware where in your moon cycle you are at all times
of the month), grounding in Nature through healthy sun exposure
and "moon baths," getting up at a regular time daily, and what I'll
spend the most time on, given this chapter's topic and the lack of
it being done, *new moon time rest*. New moon time rest is simply

the practice of doing what had been done naturally in the past in several indigenous cultures around the globe— creating protected time and space around rest during your New moon. A bit of an aside around the New moon for those who are not familiar. A woman's New moon is the time of her menstrual flow. If her cycle is regular, it is usually around every 28 days just as the moon's full orbit around the earth is also around every 28 days. The new moon in Nature is when the sky is black and the moon not visible in the sky. The full moon in Nature is of course when the moon is usually visible as a full round orb. For a woman's cycle, her Full moon is during ovulation, when she is her most fertile. There has been some literature around the importance and healthiness of a woman's New moon lining up with Nature's new moon and her Full moon lining up with Nature's full moon. Nature's new moon energetically as a woman's new moon reflects— is a time of inward, intuitive, and quiet energy. Conversely, Nature's full moon is a time of outward expression, outward connection, and creative manifestation, reflected by a woman's most fertile time, the Full moon (ovulatory) period. Syncing up one's cycle to match Nature's cycle is often thought to be beneficial and more in flow (pun entirely intended) with Nature's rhythms which prevents dis-ease in the body, especially in the womb and other sexual organs. However, there is also really interesting literature that I deeply resonate with, which offers in addition to the above, a second healthy feminine syncing with the moon[21]. In this paradigm, the woman whose cycle is aligned in the above discussed way is called a White Moon Woman but there is also a healthy alternative syncing. And it is when a woman has her New moon (her menstrual flow) during Nature's full moon and her Full Moon (ovulation) during Nature's new moon. During these times of her life, a woman is called a Red Moon Woman— and she is usually focused in her life not on procreating or birthing a child, but rather on medicinal/healing work in her community. A Red Moon woman experiences outward, creative, and healing external energy when the energy of Nature (and the community) is more inward and quiet, and then repletes her "well," so to speak, during her New moon when the energy of her environment is more expressive/creative. This makes a lot of intuitive sense to me. I wanted to offer these ideas for many women especially those who, like myself, might have felt healthy womb wise and yet felt they was something "wrong" with them because their New moon was lined up with Nature's full moon. If and when you are desiring to birth a baby, your cycle can also then shift to match Nature's cycle. I hope that is helpful to you. One last word on syncing. No matter when your menstrual flow and ovulation occur with relation to the moon, I think what's more important is that you have a healthy cycle that feels good and supportive of your best health. To encourage this, honoring the energies of the different phases of your cycle, is very helpful.

Which leads me to New moon time rest. If you are a menstruating woman, and especially if you are not in sync with the moon's cycle (whether as a White Moon or Red Moon woman), and/or if you are having irregular, painful cycles and other sexual organ symptoms, I strongly recommend that you honor the energy of your New moon. And that energy is *all* about rest. It is a time of inward energy, of the heightened intuition that comes from taking time to be still, often being alone or in quiet community with other women going through the same experience. In fact, in many indigenous communities, a gathering of the women during their new moon with an intentional retreat from the rest of the community, was a common practice. During this time, the women stayed together, supported one another, collectively harnessing the wisdom that is often brought forth from within, during these days of increased meditation and reflection. Once the New moon time was over, the women then re-entered the community with a re-centeredness and insights that supported their community. If you are a woman who is still experiencing her moon cycles, I invite you to rest more during your New moon. Rest during this time, apart from more solitude and quiet, also includes increased time away from the "screen" (TV/phones/computer) and more time with Nature. It has been my personal experience that this greatly lessens the physical and often emotional discomfort for which one's menstrual flow is notorious. Resting also means digestive rest and I have found that one's New moon time is an amazing time for doing a cleanse of some sort that resonates with you. Cleansing and shedding are literally what your body is doing during this time, through partially, the release of the uterine lining. Why not go with the flow (sorry, couldn't resist) and take advantage of the hormonal and energetic changes that promote and support physical and emotional release?

I hope some or all of the above has excited you about rest. It often gets short-thrift (if any attention at all) when we talk about health and happiness and creativity. We talk about diet and passions and what to do. I love the idea of doing LESS. Of having spaces in your day or having entire whole days as spaces without a schedule and not distracting yourself from that space with TV, social media, or even a book. In that space, I have found that there is magic waiting. There is delicious healing there and it is resting and waiting for you to join it.

My Prescription for more (and more effective) Rest:

1. Schedule in at least one 1hr (minimum) rest period this week and do it weekly for the next month. During this rest period, please do not schedule in any activity (no reading, TV watching, internet browsing, not even intentional meditation). Simply plan to do nothing.

2. During your "nothing" time, follow your intuition as to what feels good to do. Wander down a street or a path in nature, meander, lie in your bed, lounge on your back, checking out your ceiling or even better, the clouds, take a bath and just close your eyes.

3. Repeat this practice weekly for at least a month, then check in with yourself about what you have noticed from this experiment. Pay specific attention to changes in your sense of creativity, sense of feeling centered, your stress level, your interaction with others, and overall feeling of health and happiness.

Dance Link: Resting Pulses

https://www.youtube.com/watch?v=0k1XsareSCU&index=4&list=PLu5bo57nXBL34M72iL-smYfmQq1vMzVpD

CHAPTER 5

Emotion honoring and release

Darkness is a beginning

Are you feeling a storm within?
Can you stay with it a bit longer, and then
scream, sing, pray, but first do what you need
to say to it, "I hear you."

Allow it to move through your abdomen like ripe dark
berries. Let it stain your rightness like
melena. This feeling isn't a coincidence. Your weeping
has a place. Darkness is a beginning.

Let the perverse saint in you wash the feet of the
pure sinner. Take your naughty onto the dance floor.
Resistance makes the madness stronger, so
twirl instead. Try a dip or two. But try not to shrink away.

Cup the face of what you have judged as the ugly inside,
and put its whispering to your ear. And once its
voice begins to ebb, having been heard, when it slowly
fades with the dying notes of its music,
you might just find yourself humming in release, finally
healed.

-Tumi Johnson

This might be the most important chapter in the book. A bold
statement, I know, especially as the writer since each chapter of

this book is near and dear to me and chosen carefully after a lot of thought. But if I had to choose the heart of this book, it would be this one. There are a few reasons why. One, in my own personal journey of health, the ideas around this chapter that I will be sharing with you were probably the most transformative for me in not just my physical health but also my emotional well-being and sustained state of peace. Secondly, as I grow in experience as a physician, I see increasingly how the emotions of my clients and patients and the way they manage (or don't manage) them, play a potent role in their health and healing. Thirdly, this is a realm of health that I think is just not given enough attention— there is a lot of talk about what to eat, how and when to exercise, increasingly (thank goodness) on meditation and self love, but emotions? I have been to multiple medical conferences over the past two decades and this topic is not addressed. And yet, it can be the big elephant in the room, the weak link in one's health practices that makes the whole chain snap. It was for me.

Here is what happened after my suicide attempt, once I went into therapy. My disordered eating behavior quickly came out in sessions with my therapist Emily and she recommended me to group therapy with other young women who were also in the process of healing their eating issues. The group was guided by two female therapists and on the first day of our collective session, one of them gave us an unsettling instruction. She asked us that as we shared with the other group members, to refrain from talking about the food or details around the behaviors of our eating disorders, because, as she put it, "it wasn't about the food." When she said that, I remember thinking, "what do you mean it's not about the food? Why else am I here? And what am I supposed to talk about, then?" That answer became very apparent— we were invited to talk about our feelings. Even up to this point with Emily, I had spent a lot of time recounting what I had experienced as a child, a young teenager, and a young woman, but I actually hadn't spoken much about how I *felt* about these experiences. And now I was being called to do just that. And my skin started crawling. It was at that moment I realized and experienced fully this realization. It really *wasn't* about the food. The food had been the distraction for me NOT to feel what I was feeling. The food had been the drug to numb myself from feeling what I was feeling. A lot of people have read or heard about this but it's another thing to experience that reality. And you experience it when you are called to share how you feel and your skin starts crawling and words stick in your throat, and you'd rather talk/ complain about the food. And it's through that crack of discomfort that the light begins to come in. Because what I realized then is how uncomfortable I was with some of my emotions. Namely anger. I could rock joy, I could feel and express surprise very well, I had no problem embracing confusion. But with anger and all its shades (irritation, rage, and those curious zones where it crosses over into sadness, shame, and guilt), I discovered I had a hard time looking it in the eyes, much less giving it an embrace. I grew up with the teaching that anger especially from a "nice girl" wasn't pretty or kind or even palatable. And for a very long time, it was really important for me to be nice. Since I was little, I felt a strong sense of empathy for others' feelings especially when it was one of suffering and pain. It was so strong that it felt like almost too-deep sensitivity but I was told repeatedly that it just meant I was "kind," "good," "nice." And that felt good to hear, but then when other emotions outside of empathy and the desire to be kind came up— ones that were more difficult for others to take—anger for example, I was told verbally and with multiple non-verbal cues that this was not aligned with my other "better" qualities. It felt like I had to make a choice. So I held on to kind, good, nice and all their positive friends and I let go of irritation, jealousy, rage, guilt (insert other shadow emotion here). But the truth was I didn't let go of them at all. Because the reality is, the vast majority of us do not have multiple personalities. We have one whole, beautiful, and complex personality with several parts that are very much connected. Anger was a part of me and because

I couldn't face it or let it go, what I had been doing was distracting myself from it. For years. I had found methods of coping (read: disordered eating), that glazed my eyes so that I didn't have to see clearly the anger within me. I numbed myself so that I didn't have to feel its painful repeated pinching. And the more I numbed myself, the more I could project the positive parts of myself and hide the parts of myself, including emotions, that others and now myself had judged as "bad." And all the while, the distraction, the numbing, the pushing down of these emotions were making me sicker and sicker until I found myself in that hospital bed. Because, here's the kicker, the eureka insight that changed my emotional life, not to mention my path and philosophical practice as a healer: those "bad" emotions, if we pay attention to them, are just as much our friends, our guides, our teachers, as the "good" emotions. In fact, at times, more so. They can give us *very* good information about what is not healthy in our lives. Here is what I learned about anger (this is the emotion I present as an example because it was my most prominent shadow or "difficult" emotion). Anger was pinching at my elbow even as I tried swiping it away from touching me (with numbing food), to let me know that there were some seriously messed up dynamics in my core relationships that were not healthy for me, and needed changing ASAP. I've read somewhere that often when you feel anger, it can be good information that you have let your healthy boundaries be breached. And this was definitely the case with me. A few healthy boundaries had been breached; some had not been properly erected in the first place. And anger was calling my attention to it. But I didn't want to look. Apart from feeling the emotion I had judged as bad, looking at the problem and truly feeling my emotion would also mean I would have to change things. And change can feel very, very scary.

A brief aside about change— it has been my experience that all seven of the healing aspects in this book have also helped me navigate change with so much more grace than ever before in my life, especially the aspect of self love (talked about in the last chapter).

In terms of *how* I learned to look anger in the eye, it was really helpful for me to hear that anger was on my side, that it wasn't a monstrous emotion that I should avoid, fight, or "conquer" in order to be my best self. That in fact anger, like any emotion I felt, was in service to me, helping me to be my best, truest self. And to really take that in, I had to learn that there was a difference between feeling my emotions and acting out those emotions. I also had to recognize that there was a space in between the two (the feeling and the action). And this was a space that made ALL the difference in whether feeling anger resulted in my positive growth and healing, or whether it resulted in my suffering. It is that space I would like to devote time to in this chapter.

This is the space in which emotion honoring and release can occur. It is a healing space and one I guide a lot of clients and patients into, after having spent a lot of time exploring and mastering that space myself.

So what happens in this space? What does emotion honoring and release look like? It starts with the emotion felt and then everything from there on, is your choice. You can choose to look at the emotion and acknowledge it, or run screaming in the other direction and try to snuff it out then bury your emotion with a distracting, numbing activity of your selection (there are many choices for this). Here are the steps I have developed to create the most positive and healing outcome. I have clarified and honed these steps myself over years but I would like to thank Veronica Krestow and her Diamond Process[1] for being helpful to me in crafting some of these steps!

1. When the difficult emotion appears, rather than avoiding it, stop what you are doing and take the time to look at it

in the eyes like you would a friend. Do this especially if it's a difficult emotion because it means your teacher, healer, physician has arrived. Practically, this looks like carving out some space in your day as soon as you can to "be" with this emotion rather than distracting yourself from it.

2. Take this friend/teacher's hands into yours and feel its touch. In other words, *feel the emotion.* Observe where on or in your body you feel sensations, where things clench or release, sink or elevate, twist, turn, vibrate. Allow yourself to feel all of this. This is part of crucial information gathering, of listening to the lesson being given. Also, please try to do this with as little judgment as possible. Remember the space: the feelings and thoughts DON'T translate to your actions directly. So allow yourself to experience them without the fear that you are a bad person for the thought/feeling and that it doesn't have to result in you becoming a violent human being (for example, in the case of anger).

3. Speaking of fear, ask yourself what fears are coming up for you around this difficult emotion. As the saying goes, fear is false expectations appearing real. So explore the fear based false ideas or assumptions that are coming up for you with this emotion. I'll give you a specific example: say you feel anger when your partner forgets your birthday. The fear-based false idea around this might be "I am no longer a lovable human being" or "I am clearly forgettable if my own partner doesn't remember an important occasion." As you may have noticed, these statements have nothing to do with your partner. Maybe it's not a false idea that she/he doesn't love you. But what definitely *is* false is that you are not lovable. So I invite you during these steps to make the statements about yourself and not any other person. It is empowering to do this because you can take responsibility for yourself and not for anyone else's feelings or actions. I have found that it is helpful for me to write out these false

statements on paper. When I see their words, they lose their power in a big sense (as they can often be a source of shame if we feel scared to speak or write them out). Doing the above both honors our emotions as well as releases them from our bodies either verbally or through the cathartic process of writing.

4. After doing the above, with a whole lot of compassion, you then tell yourself positive, loving and self-affirming statements that address the fear-based untruths or assumptions from step 3. In the case of above, it would look like "I am lovable as I am" or "I am someone worth remembering (we all are)."

5. Finally I ask myself, "what is the lesson here? Though this difficult emotion that is coming up, what is asking to be healed?" In the example above, it might be a request for more self-love. If your self-love tank were full, your partner forgetting your birthday would not bother you as much. On a side note, if she/he doesn't love you, that self love could also be the engine to guide you away from a relationship that is lacking in love.

6. The final and important step is gratitude for the emotion, even as it fades away as the lesson has been learnt. That has been my experience over and over again: as I glean wisdom from the emotions I am feeling, the emotion, having done its work, calmly leaves.

So how does this translate into real life? I'll offer my personal experience as an example. In the past, when I felt a difficult emotion, my immediate question was "how can I make this go away as soon as possible?" Enter in binge eating. Now when I feel a difficult emotion, my first question is "why is this happening FOR me?" As is detailed in the first step of emotion honoring/release, recognition of our emotions as our warriors, as occurring to *help* us, is so crucial in resisting the urge to squelch the said emotion. My past initial question and response was based in fear. My question and response now are mired in self-confidence. Confidence that parts of my self (including the difficult emotions) are on my side and show up to teach and heal me.

To be clear, when these emotions are honored and released, they don't necessarily go away forever. Anger has come up time and time again and each time, it has something to teach me. The goal is *not* to get rid of our difficult emotions "once and for all" by doing the above practice. Rather, it is to realize again, that our emotions are on our side to show us something important that is asking to be addressed in our lives. Now you might be thinking, "practically, doing all the above each time I have a difficult emotion just doesn't make a lot of sense. I'd be 'honoring/releasing' all day and wouldn't be able to get anything done!" My experience has been that emotions usually have different intensities. You will not have to think about the "lesson of the emotion" for every nuanced difficult emotion you feel. What I invite you to do though, is to allow yourself to acknowledge, even welcome in, all the emotions you *do* feel throughout the day. Sometimes that is all the emotion needs and wants from you. Sometimes though, it wants more, and you'll know when, because likely you'll feel a bit overwhelmed or a lot overwhelmed by it. That one, that level of intensity, is the one to look at closely when you've carved time out later that day and do the above limned exercise. Speaking of which, yes, I recommend that anytime you feel a strong difficult emotion intensely, to do most/all of the above steps that same day. There's wisdom to that old adage of not going to bed angry. In my observation, the practice of "storing away" day after day any difficult emotion, until some future time when it's convenient for you, almost always backfires.

Also, one tip that I would like to offer has to do with the moment you might feel any intense emotion. It is not always convenient when it happens. In fact, oftentimes, intense emotions don't appear when you are in the sanctuary of your home or some other safe and isolated place. They can occur at first dates, at company meetings, at weddings, on a public bus. This does not mean that these situations give us liberty to then numb or distract ourselves from the emotion, so that we don't look crazy or turn into a "puddle" in front of strangers. Remember again that our emotions are on our side and don't come up to sabotage us. You might think your emotion is telling you for example, "Oh you like this girl do you? Hmm. Well here comes jealousy but don't feel it, buddy, because then she's going to see just how crazy you are." No, that's not how it works. In fact, as mentioned above, I think it's *not* allowing yourself to feel the jealousy, the shame, the pettiness, etc, that results in others "seeing just how crazy you are." And that happens when all that repressed emotion explodes at some point. And it always explodes. Or implodes.

But yes, it is not always an opportune time to steep yourself in the feeling and do the above exercises I described above. So then what? Here's what I suggest and have practiced and continue to practice with success. This wisdom comes from yoga, and it is called pratyahara. It is the practice of intentionally withdrawing one's senses from the external situation at hand. I've heard it described as a turtle withdrawing a little bit into his shell. It does not have to be a complete "disappearing act" in which you are no longer engaging with the people you might have been talking with, but it can be rather, a slight pull back. A lot of times, especially in emotionally charged events, we can tend to "over-engage" and over-extend ourselves emotionally in the situation. We are holding our breath, we aren't breaking eye contact, we are even possibly leaning forward physically in the interaction. There are no pauses in the conversation. Now if this is happening naturally and feels good, wonderful. We've all been there, in a flow of conversation and attraction and connection with another human being or other human beings, and it is beautiful. But. There are also situations in which one person is doing all the work of connecting (or attempting to connect) and providing emotional support, while the other person is soaking it up, intentionally or otherwise. Here is a hint: a good way to know if you are giving way too much emotionally in an interaction is *after* the interaction— if you are feeling fatigued, emotionally depleted, irritated, resentful (again, emotions as very good teachers), this might be you. Or say it is a mutual and wonderful exchange and then all of a sudden, here comes "difficult emotion." In both situations, pratyahara is a great practice. Step back a little: this might look like breaking eye contact a bit, taking a few slow deep breaths, leaning back. It may even look like asking to be excused and taking a moment literally away from the situation. I am astounded when I look back at my life prior to this practice, how many times I would literally just stay in really unpleasant conversations and situations, fully engaged, rather than exercising a little self-care and leaving. Pratyahara offers the choice of mindful, subtle leaving. Or maybe, better put, returning. Returning to the home of your body, your breath, your self. And there, you can embrace that difficult emotion with a kind acknowledgment, prepare a seat for him, tell him you'll be back, and then go back to the outside world until you have time alone later to converse and learn from him.

And now for some words of assurance: this all gets easier. It gets so much easier. The first few days and perhaps weeks doing the above steps consistently with your emotions might feel slightly painful and even tedious. As an aside, I personally never found it tedious because the lessons from these exercises that I received were never boring. But it can feel raw because you're allowing yourself to feel. Please trust the process.

Part of the process, I must add, is honing this release practice. Meaning that after crafting what seems like a good emotion honoring/release practice for yourself, and starting to do it consistently, there is almost always "relapse." Relapse in this context, looks like reverting to any activity (usually your old favorites) to numb out the difficult emotion that comes up. During my psychosocial training in medical residency, I learned that relapse is an often under-appreciated and misunderstood step of permanent and positive behavioral change. You can choose to think of relapse as failure, but if you do so, you've missed the point and worse, your self-esteem has suffered because of the choice. Or, you can choose to think of relapse as fantastic information. Anytime a patient of mine tells me they've "relapsed," I rub my palms together excitedly and lean forward and ask "tell me exactly what happened" like a tween about to get a juicy story from her best friend. And that's because the story is ripe with potential pearls. That which bumped you off the proverbial wagon is exactly the thing you need to master to stay on the wagon the next time. So concretely, if someone told me that after just three days of their crafted emotion honoring/release practice, they were back to numbing out, and that FYI, those three days were pure torture, then usually that tells me that they need to change what they are doing for their practice. If someone however tells me that it was going great for three *weeks,* then they skipped on doing one part of their practice and two days later, they found themselves eating an entire pizza so as not to feel sad, that is also good information. It tells me that the part of their practice they skipped out on, is a crucial daily practice. I think you get the point. If you relapse, simply get back on the wagon but now doing something differently— tweaking your strategy. And keep doing this until you are not clutching to the sides of the wagon, but you are now coasting and enjoying the ride and the view. And trust me, it will happen.

What I can share with you now after emerging from the "other side," after diving deep and creating a practice of looking at, sitting with, and learning from my emotions, is that not only does the practice of this get easier, I feel an overall much increased feeling of emotional resilience. I still feel strongly about a lot of things, but because I now have a practice of welcoming those feelings, those feelings don't cling on, digging their fingers in my arms because they know they are about to be shaken off violently, or treated poorly. Instead, being welcomed, they embrace me briefly, whisper their wisdom, and then are off.

If all this seems sort of hazy and abstract, cloaked in too many metaphors, my only advice is to just try it yourself. Do this if this issue of emotion honoring and release is a weak point for you (and I believe from my experience, it is a weak point for many). In fact, I believe it to be one of the key reasons for persistent addictions of all kinds and as you practice the above, what I have shared will quickly become very real and concrete for you. And when it does, remember this: "darkness is a beginning." Remember to "cup the face of what you have judged as the ugly inside, and put its whispering to your ear. And once its voice begins to ebb, having been heard, when it slowly fades with the dying notes of its music, you might just find yourself humming in release, finally healed."

My Prescription for creating your unique emotion honoring/release practice:

Ask yourself the following 4 questions:

1. *What emotions do I usually try to suppress with distracting or numbing activities?*
2. *What activities, if any, do I do regularly to check in with my emotions? (examples include meditation, journaling, therapy, or open talk with a trusted loved one)*
3. *Which activities, if any, help me feel like I have truly "released" my emotions, especially the above ones from question 1? (examples include journaling, physical movement, healthy vocalization)*
4. *What activities, if any, help me feel like I'm truly grounded and connected with myself? (examples include time in Nature, singing, meditation, art, prayer, capoeira etc).*

If you find that you often suppress your emotions, try increasing or implementing more of the activities from your answers to questions 2-4.

Dance Link: Darkness is a Beginning

https://www.youtube.com/watch?v=sJOgGvh8hig

CHAPTER 6

Nature

Finally fall

At first, I thought bats but I was in downtown Brooklyn but then again, it had been a strange September. At the second strike against the windowpane, I saw a flash of sly color.
Curlicues of fiber making their way to asphalt through any means necessary. Slow showers of stiff cut paper. The tree was shaking the beads off her wrists, and here they were going down, suicidal birds pirouetting past my eye like brilliant scotomas.

Last night, I pressed myself against the corner of the closet door frame, closed my eyes and it was as though you were here, matching my light.
The leaves, like me, take on the hue of a slow burn. With my lips against old white wood, I whispered like a season turning, beckoned like a girl made newly into woman, *love,*
Love.

- Tumi Johnson

A significant part of this book was written in Bali and I feel so grateful to be writing this chapter on Nature here in one of the most stunning places I've ever been to on this earth. The green of the rice fields after the rain is a shade of green I've never seen in natural colors. The pops of red from the flowers peeking from trees and the sheer abundance of lushness offered by Nature—all of this greet my eyes in the morning and have been the perfect backdrop to write this chapter.

My boyfriend and I spent two months in our beautiful jungle-like abode about eight miles outside of Ubud, surrounded by frangipani, as well as banana, papaya, and moringa trees. There were crickets to sing us to sleep and roosters to rouse us from it (although in truth, they bellowed all day not just in the morning). Geckos studded our walls and the high rafters of the ceiling and lay out with us on the porch. We ate in the sun, slapping at the mosquitos, and my daily dance class was often on the bare grass. And for whole days and sometime two day stretches, especially during the downpours of rain, we didn't leave our tropical space to venture out to the city. And the lessons from this time have been incredible. Here are some of what I experienced and what I learned from this beautiful place.

1. Nature is very good at upturning one's plans. If you thought I was going to start these lessons with something fluffier or sweeter, nope. This was one of the first reminders I had being in Bali. It rained, as in *poured*, for four days straight. On the first day, I cheerfully put on my too bright orange rain jacket and splashed through the streets of Ubud in sandals, ducking under temple awnings to taste new fruit. On the second day, I less cheerfully donned on said rain jacket. On the third day without any glimpse of sunlight, just persistent rain, I sat behind the mosquito nets on our bed and peered out morosely at the weather. And we had to do some serious re-arranging of plans. My dance classes got moved indoors since the porch was soaked and too slippery to dance on. Our ideas of exploring the town by walking or biking were put aside. By the fourth day, I was feeling a strong sense of annoyance and was reminded how in some ways, I am not so much a free spirit. This feeling invited me to look at where my anger was coming from (see the last chapter), and what this feeling was teaching me. And here was the lesson: "Let go. Make your plans if you like, if it makes you feel calmer and more in control, but make them

loosely, because you never know." It is a lesson, in short, of presence. Of dis-attachment from the outcome, from the un-real future. I can share with you that one of the times I am most present is hiking uphill in a bug-ridden forest. Between the buzz of flies to which I'm hypersensitive, and the ever-changing underground with rocks, brambles and perhaps a low lying creature, not to mention the actual exercise, my mind really doesn't tend to wander anywhere being fully occupied with the sensorial input of the now. Nature often offers this— swimming in an ocean with large waves is another example for me. Your mind will not wander watching and preparing for those waves. Furthermore, with regards to Nature's lesson in "making plans loosely," it is not a lesson of being flaky or giving up what you love. Nature wasn't telling me "it's raining, sorry you can't dance." Instead it was saying, "it's raining, there isn't sun, NOW what do you feel like dancing to, and *how* do you feel like dancing? And here, try dancing indoors again for once." In other words, it offers the very beautiful option of getting more flexible, of being creative, of learning how to be resilient. Rather than fighting against the situation, there is the opportunity to look at what is happening beyond your control and then decide on how it can be "for you." If that reframing feels completely out of the question (there are some days/ situations in which you may not be willing to ask yourself that question), then rather, ask "how can I stay present to this?" or "What is it teaching me?" and (a wonderful one for us all to keep practicing), "how can I release just a little more, the noose of my plans, become less rigid, and let go of the illusion of control." Crazy transformative things start happening when you make this choice. This has been my experience. To pull from another tropical metaphor, I think the difference is comparing a concrete building to a bamboo one. The concrete building, which though solid is rigid, has the tendency to feel stuffy and mold in hot wet climates. In contrast, bamboo is breathable and flexible. Resilient, it can bend with the storms but maintains its integrity. Which would you prefer to be? Working with patients and clients, I often see those who come in with an "all or nothing" philosophy about health and their health behaviors, who "fight" against circumstances that are out of their control, and feel they are at "war" with their bodies or in a constant struggle to "achieve health." These are the ones who have the hardest time getting to and maintaining their best well-being. One of the reasons I love my work as a doctor is guiding people in navigating through the very real life situations while maintaining the integrity of their health intentions and purposes. A key pearl I try to impart, is that rather than trying to fight, rather than thinking that Nature and circumstance are against you and out plotting your health demise, to recognize instead that Nature just *is*. Circumstance just *is*. It is your response that determines your reality, and it is your mental state that shifts your response. Here is another truth/lesson about Nature to help keep one's mental state in a place that allows you to feel and respond with your true power:

2. We ARE Nature. We are a part of the crazy, mystical, powerful beauty and mystery of what Nature is. We may have forgotten that, in all our tales of "us versus Nature, but" those are fear- based and stem from self-limiting paradigms. Here is another and in my opinion, truer tale: we are just another element of Nature, like stones, trees, a deer, an eagle, the wide ocean. And all of these elements influence us, just as we influence them. In our en masse movements into cities and away from more natural environments, with our erections of more and more artificial structures and our ripping out of some of our oldest wisest elders, Trees, we may have forgotten that truth. But our body remembers: when

rain approaches and our joints tell us so, the way a woman's menstrual cycle is in rhythm with the moon, the way our breaths get slower and deeper, our spines lift, and visions clear along with our minds when we are in what we call "Nature." When we recognize ourselves as a part of Nature, as holding within us the very elements of Nature itself, we begin to honor the cycles within our body and lives better, and I think that puts us in greater synchronicity, synergy, and thus effort-less well-being. One beautiful practice I now love doing while in Nature is to ask it something, ask a question with which I am grappling. And then just get still. The answer in some form or the other, always comes. To me this is further evidence of the Divine in Nature, us as a part of Nature and thus, the Divine within us. For as we ask the question, we are really approaching Spirit. And as we get quiet, we hear the answer from that still small voice within, the voice that is also contained in the bark of the tree we touch, in the sea in which we have immersed ourselves, the rock in our palm.

3. Nature will bring up your stuff. You know—that stuff that you buried so deep that you sometimes forgot it was a thing, except in quiet moments which you have crowded out with any busy activity you can come up with. There is a great poem by John Muir that rephrased states that by going out in Nature, we are often going within ourselves. Many people have a hard time with that which is why people often flee from Nature. I had a patient who would tell me stories of going very often to the woods because he constantly felt pulled there (as we all do in some way to Nature). However, upon returning, he would inevitably get plastered drunk, more so than when he stayed *out of* Nature. Your stuff that comes up can look like many things. I mentioned previously my hypersensitivity to flies. It is something that is now getting better but in the past, it is often the reason

I would identify myself as a "nature lover" but without the confident perky tone. If there was a fly in the room, I was very aware of it. And not happy about it. I've apparently had this aversion since I was a young child in West Africa and all my years of yoga and meditation, while they have greatly eased the discomfort around flies, have not eradicated it. During my first ten day Vipassana silent meditation course in the Joshua Tree dessert of California, I was day five out of ten in, feeling in general pretty proud of myself. I felt like I was doing pretty well (i.e. not running for the hills, or in this case, back to L.A. after five days each consisting of 10 hours of meditation, and 24 hours of pure silence and no eye contact with no allowed yoga or dancing even in my room). I was about 50 minutes into an hour long meditation, in which it is invited to practice strong determination and not move one's limbs. I was feeling a little cocky about how easy this was all getting, and then the buzz hit my left ear. That frequency and sound that could only be from *Musca domestica*, known commonly as a fly. I can tell you that the last 10 minutes of that meditation were probably some of the longest of my entire life. My skin was crawling, I felt itchy and I wanted to run screaming from the room. "Over a fly?" You might ask. Well insert your phobia here and you will get it. I have taken long luscious showers with walls full of spiders and large lizards. I have survived a scorpion bite and didn't think to change my sleeping quarters where the undiscovered scorpion rested. I grew up with cobras in my backyard and daydreamed comfortably in the grass for several hours. But flies? Not a fan. We all have our thing. It is the thing that keeps us humble. My cockiness at the meditation course was cured from that moment on. Each time after, when I entered that meditation hall and closed my eyes to begin the mindfulness practice, I knew there was a chance for that buzz to return and so my practice of presence up-leveled to a whole new degree. We all have our thing. And Nature often will bring it to you. Nature can stir up a lot of discomfort because it often will excavate your dis-ease and bring it up to the surface. However by doing so, it offers up incredible healing potential. To be ready for that— to choose to use the discomfort as a gift rather than to quell it by any means possible, please see my previous chapters on meditation as well as emotion honoring.

These are my experiential lessons from Nature. And no surprise, scientific literature affirms that Nature does a body (and mind) good. Really good.

In a study published in Psychologic Science, a group of University of Michigan students were administered a memory test then divided into two groups. One group then took a walk around an arboretum while the other group took a walk down a city street. When the participants returned and repeated the test, it was found that the group who had been in the arboretum performed almost 20% better than their first test; the group that had taken in the city sights did not improve their scores[1]. Another study also looking at Nature's effect on memory and published in the Journal of Affective Disorders, found that nature walks boosted working memory of depressed individuals much more than walks in urban environments[2]. Speaking of mood, there have also been studies that show a significant improvement of anxiety and depression after exposure to Nature, especially forest walks[3,4,5]. One study, published in the Proceedings of the National Academy of Science[6], found that individuals walking for 90 minutes in a natural setting, compared to participants walking in a high-traffic urban environment, exhibited decreased activity in an area of the brain associated with a key factor in depression. Specifically, brain activity in the subgenual prefrontal cortex, a region active during rumination (repetitive thought focused on negative emotions), decreased significantly among the study participants who walked in the natural environment compared to those who walked in the urban setting. There are studies that also suggest that a prescription of "Nature" can be quite helpful for treating ADHD in children[7,8].

Science has demonstrated that the positive effects of Nature extend past our brain and nerve health. An intriguing study from Japan looked at the immune response of a group of women who over the course of two days, spent six hours in the woods. The study investigators found that these women after this exposure in Nature, had an increase in virus- and tumor-fighting white blood cells, with this positive effect lasting for at least seven days after their time in Nature[9].

Also, inflammation, a hot target of both mainstream and more "alternative" forms of medical treatment, has been shown to also be relieved by exposure to Nature. Cortisol is an increasingly spoken about hormone because it is often used as a marker of chronic stress, and overproduction can instigate and exacerbate inflammation in the body. Studies have now found lower levels of cortisol in those who spend time in Nature versus those who do not[10,11].

So those are just a few of the studies. And the next obvious question is "how?" How does one "connect more with nature?" This might not seem evident especially if you consider yourself more of a "city mouse" and/or the idea of camping or hiking in Nature already causes you to break out in hives. And even those of us who consider ourselves to be "nature lovers" (with or without the perky tone) can always benefit from deepening our connection with Nature. As a generalization, the vast majority of us are much removed (in varying degrees) from this connection. I think on a side note, this might be a reason for Western society's fairly new obsession with post-apocalyptic TV shows and movies. I think there is a real understanding that many of us are disconnected from Nature (in several senses of that word). There is a hunger not just to know that one could survive if all our luxuries were taken and we were left on the side of the mountain, but a hunger to perhaps experience some of that. So— how?

I don't think it has to be as dramatic as the scenarios play out on the screen, or you having to decide to make a trek through the Himalayas to re-connect with Nature (although if that is what is calling to you, then that's great). Like most things, consistent and regular exposure even in small doses is often much more potent than very occasional and inconsistent exposure. An example of this would be hiking daily in the woods or swimming in a nearby stream having more of health benefit over time than once every few years, taking a one week trip to the mountains and the rest of the time, having little engagement with Nature.

If your response is that there are no woods nor nearby clean streams available to you, I want to remind you of the preceding chapters in which Nature was "snuck" into other things. Here are some simple but powerful ways of deepening your connection with Nature, pulled from the previous chapters and expounded upon here.

The first (from Chapter 1) is to eat more real food. More food that comes from Nature. Food that is unpackaged, unprocessed, that is vibrant with natural colors and the nutrients from Mama Earth. Whole fruits and vegetables, preferably in season. The food we choose to eat is one of our most powerful connections with Nature. We literally take in more Nature when we eat let's say a ripe Honeycrisp apple in the autumn or a beautifully fresh watermelon in the height of summer. We affirm that we ARE Nature when we do this in a way that eating a bowl of frosted mini wheats or having a donut just does not. When we then compost the left-overs of said real food and even better, plant those apple or watermelon seeds, we are helping with that circle of life and giving back to Nature in a very palpable way. Being conscious and intentional about our food choices, about selecting foods whose journey to your table left a lighter "footprint" on the earth, is one of greatest things you can do to feel that connection with Nature. And as more and more evidence demonstrates, the lightest footprint comes from us eating plants — especially fruits and all preferably locally grown. If you are a city mouse, living in a city with farmers' markets, I can share with you that during my ten years in New York City, a regular trip to the farmer's market was very centering for me. I think that this is because it's not just about eating this great food, it's about seeing it in its most natural form, touching it, speaking to those who have grown it. Planting is another really wonderful way of feeling that connection, especially if you live in a city and/or food desert. Growing greens and herbs inside your living space is so gratifying, grounding, and further fosters that connection with Nature. There are an increasing number of inspiring people living in food deserts and inner cities and yet acting as pioneers and starting community gardens in their neighborhoods[12].

Other ways of connecting to Nature no matter where you live are through sun-gazing and moon watching. Sun-gazing has been a practice done for centuries. Moon watching is something I began doing a few years ago when I wanted to track my menstrual cycle and naturally regulate it. Being aware of the cycles of the moon and their respective different energies is beneficial for both men and women. However, if you are a woman who is menstruating, it is my opinion that this awareness as well as simple practices that respect the different energies throughout the moon cycle, can be amazingly beneficial for not just regulating one's cycle but also healing menstrual discomfort (both physically and emotionally).

Other ways of deepening connection with Nature include having natural elements of Nature inside your home— I have mentioned plants already. These can be edible or not. Also, having and lighting candles and fireplaces (fire is a powerful element of Nature), having art that depicts Nature as well as having around elements of Nature that you may have collected from a trip (example: rocks, crystals, shells). Doing this with your living space is a great reminder of that irrevocable connection and your true identity as a Nature being.

If you do have Natural beauty accessible to you— whether it's a woody trail, a city park, a waterfall, a mountain, spend as much time in/on/near it as possible. And I recommend doing it throughout the seasons. I can share that the winter in New York City I started running outdoors as part of my exercise, was the winter I stopped fearing and dreading that season, and feeling so cold during it. Spending considerable time in Nature during the different seasons helps our bodies acclimate to the changes. We become "inoculated" by Dr. Mother Gaia. I mentioned before in Chapter 2 that I believe Nature to provide the best fitness course and so I recommend whenever possible, doing one's movement practice in Nature. Also incorporating your rest and meditative practices with time in Nature is synergistic and I highly suggest it. So rather than reading this chapter and thinking, "Oh here's another thing I have to do— spend time in Nature," this is one realm in which I encourage you to multi-task. When you can, eat in Nature, move in Nature, rest in Nature, meditate in Nature. I think you get the point. The more we do these practices in alignment with Nature, through these small but powerful gestures, the more we feel that connection with Nature that is our reality but which many of us have forgotten. And then, something truly profound begins to happen— a sense of wholeness and connectedness begins to grow. You recognize that as part of Nature and with the power that you wield, and with the beauty and healing she provides, that you can be a steward of the Earth. This consciousness has been so heart opening for me: to recognize that my actions from the food I eat, to the way I consume in general, what I spend my money on, how I travel, how I speak and move in the world, has ripple-like consequences that affect the many species and biomes of our planet. And THAT has consequences on my life and the lives of those I love. In brief, we are all connected, and Nature is one of the best teachers for this. The very experiential knowledge of that inter-connectedness offers a sense of wholeness. Wholeness. The very definition of healing.

My Prescription for deepening your sense of connection with Nature:

1. Bring in elements of Nature into each room of your home/ living space. This might be a candle that you light regularly, an arrangement of seashells, a piece of wood or a crystal. Touch these items regularly to feel that irrevocable tie you have with the earth.

2. Think of one way in which you can increase your time spent in Nature on a weekly (if not daily basis). If time pressed, consider one of the health activities presented in previous chapters and consider doing it in a Nature setting (example: your movement practice, meditation, eating a meal). Schedule this time in Nature (rather than just thinking you'd like to do it) in your calendar and do this at least weekly (if not daily).

3. Ask yourself "how can I become a better steward of the earth?" and choose an activity to begin doing something that better supports the health of our planet. This might be choosing a more plant based diet, it might be recycling or re-using more, switching from plastic to re-usable bags. Choose an activity and give yourself a 30 day challenge to do this activity. Doing it for 30 days can then motivate you to continue this new positive activity indefinitely. Remember the health of this planet is strongly connected to your own well-being.

Dance Link: I Am The Sane

https://www.youtube.com/watch?v=p_FdKjbCJHQ&t=25s

CHAPTER 7

Love

Shed the Head

Is love our vestige? We walk with the shrunken
remains of it, trying to hide it
like an unsatisfactory appendage,
like a fin. What are the apertures to our oldest selves?—
kindness, tears, unadulterated
joy? Silence is being replaced by
any noise we can make. And we
are making it loudly, deafening the present.
What are the undiscovered folds of the brain?
Tucked into their recesses is a reassurance.
We are from the same tribe.

But love has been quoted into gradiations
Degraded into quotients. As we make the cut,
Somehow none of us is making the cut. How does one
shed the head?

If you forget everything, remember this:
You have a place at the table.
Remember that the most important memory
is right now and was always right now.
Forget it. The memory is gone.
Can you remember this?:

Yes.

- Tumi Johnson

Please don't mistake my placement of this chapter in the book as a reflection that I prioritize all the other aspects of healing as higher than love. If anything, it was very clear to me when creating this book that I wanted to end with Love because it is this that I want most fresh, most powerfully in your mind when you finish this book. In short, I saved the best for last.

There are countless stories, poems, and songs written about love and they are done in the most different appearing cultures and traditions. And that is because love is part of what makes us human. Love is universal, it connects, it transcends, and it heals. You probably know of at least one person past or present who seemed to be doing everything wrong health-wise: maybe they smoked, drank too much, and ate nothing I recommended in Chapter 1, and yet they lived long lives. And it's absolutely befuddling and a bit maddening to many an earnest health-seeker. Well before reaching for burgers and fries and saying "so and so did this and lived a long life," remember love. For me, the goal is not to support you in just living long but for however long you do live, to live happily *and* healthily and the two are intertwined. If the person you are thinking of lived long, healthily AND happily, that person was probably very much in love. That is to say, the person was steeped in love, love was a guiding principle and practice in his or her life, whether consciously or not. Love guided that person in his or her choices, in interactions with others. It was the barometer for a good life.

And when I mean love, I don't mean love limited to love of a romantic partner or a child or a pet. It might be love of music, of sport, of one's work/calling, it might be love of Nature, love of animals. One of these loving relationships may have been a "portal" to someone's experience of Love but my point is that it's all the same. What is important is the vibration that is felt from that relationship. And it is a vibration of connection, of wholeness, of expansiveness. It is a vibration of unlimitedness, of peace, complete and pure joy. This vibration is really important to understand as the feeling of true love and it is the way I would ask oneself if the "connection" one is feeling is love or not. You might say, "I really LOVE shopping but when I do it, I don't feel expansive or whole nor at peace; and often when I don't do it, I feel very anxious, and I tend to feel guilty. And I wouldn't say that my shopping habit makes me happy overall." That's not love. It is an unhealthy attachment and might be addiction and it's important to recognize it as such. Please see more of healing addiction in Chapter 5.

Again, I believe true love, no matter its form or specific relationship, feels like expansiveness, empathy, connection. It is, to dumb it down, *positive.* And this is what I feel from anyone with whom I work who has love in his or her life in a very significant and consistent way.

How do you recognize someone in love? And I speak not about those who have "fallen" in "love" but rather have "climbed up" to it, those who have welcomed it and have chosen it, again and again. In my experience, those in this state of love are the people who emanate a feeling of peace. A feeling of acceptance, compassion, and goodwill. And to be clear, it is not about being perfect. When we think of models of love in both secular and Spiritual realms- say MLK Jr, Ghandi, Jesus, Mother Theresa, the Buddha, none of this individuals were without the very human emotions of anger, fear, shame, doubt, as stories of them reflect. However, these names repeatedly come up when one thinks of Love, because for many, through their actions, they showed that Love was their guiding principle.

And if that all seems just gushy and you'd like to hear some palpable evidence for Love being good for your health, here are a few.

1) A meta-analysis study published in Health Psychology[1] showed that self-compassion (accepting yourself without judgment) is linked to better health behaviors. This analysis

looked at fifteens studies of more than 3,000 people across the age spectrum, and discovered a strong correlation between self-compassion and four key health-promoting behaviors: eating better, exercising more, getting more restful sleep, and stressing less. People who were more self-compassionate practiced these health habits more often. The potency of these health habits and the diseases that can occur when we don't engage in them (heart disease, diabetes, obesity, chronic pain, cancer, to name just a few) is well known, and has been discussed in previous chapters.

2) I think that the work of Dr. Kristin Neff around self compassion is really note-worthy. Dr. Neff, an associate professor of human development at the University of Texas at Austin has done significant research showing that those with high levels of self-compassion fair better than those with self-described high self-esteem in terms of weathering anxiety-provoking situations and nurturing well-being[2].

3) Self-love, it seems is also crucial when recovering from a broken heart. Logical, but also backed by science. In a study published in Psychological Science, researchers found that newly divorced people who spoke compassionately toward themselves adjusted significantly better, in the following 9 months, with self-compassion being as a good predictor of healthy emotional coping[3].

4) Love and its health benefits stretch beyond self-love. A study published in the International Journal of Psychophysiology demonstrated that people who gave social support to others had lower blood pressure than people who didn't. It appeared that the supportive interaction with others also helped people recover from heart disease-related events. The study researchers also discovered that those who were involved in helping others through community and organizational involvement, had greater self-esteem, less depression and lower stress levels than those who didn't[4].

5) The health benefits of altruism are well studied and the following study is yet another one that supports the above findings. This one found that older residents of California who volunteered in two or more organizations were 44 percent lower mortality (less likely to die) than people who didn't volunteer! The study accounted for other factors including age, exercise practices, and unhealthy habits such as smoking.[5]

Hopefully I have convinced you (if you needed convincing) of why love is integral to your health. And now, the question might be, "how do I 'get' love, keep love, and grow it?" And I think that is a fantastic question. Just as we spent time talking about how to craft a meditation practice and a movement play practice, I believe it is vital to talk about how to cultivate a love practice. My philosophy about love, at least the love that I speak of here, is that it is not limited to a feeling but actually is a *practice* which then nurtures and expands a feeling. Just like the right movement play practice for you will nurture and expand feelings of fitness, and literally up your feel-good hormones, the practice of love nurtures and expands feelings of empathy, goodwill, peace, and harmony, all of which, as discussed above, are amazing for your health, the health of others, and of our world.

So how do we get, keep, and nurture love? It has been my experience that it begins with your Self. Not the smaller case "s" but the big letter "S," The S that connects us with Spirit, that recognizes that we are greater than the limits of our body and often our thoughts. And furthermore, it has been my experience that the the love of Self intertwines with the love of others as well the love of Spirit/the Divine. That is the nature of Love. It doesn't know when to stop. It is limitless. And it is true that when one approaches one aspect of love, all other aspects are positively affected. But. There are some mistruths and imbalances I have seen, especially in the societies in which I was raised, that can often skew one's idea of love.

Let me get specific. There are a LOT of love songs about loving someone, about not being able to "breathe" without the person. How one can't "live if living is without you," etcetera. Simply listen to some of the most popular love songs and start paying attention to how much self-annihilation is present in the lyrics. Even when the singer is purportedly happy and so "in love," there is a genuine lack of self awareness. And trust me, I get it. I have "fallen in love" so hard that it takes my breath away and all the cheesiest of songs suddenly make absolute sense to me. But I think what comes after, the actual relationship is what bears looking at. Is it one in which you love the other, are loved by the other, and in which you feel self love? That, I would offer is true love— expansive, freeing, and healthy. If the relationship stays tortured with you breathless, feeling ungrounded, quaking in your shoes (and months or years later, you keep telling yourself it's a thrill not fear), then you might need to take a closer look at that relationship. And I think the best way to do that is often through looking at your relationship with yourself.

The remedy that took me from a frightened, disconnected, and hope-less young woman on that hospital bed more than 15 years ago to the woman I am today involved a big dose of self love. And that did not come so readily. In general, we are not given a lot encouragement to love ourselves unconditionally. Rather, we are told in many different arenas (school, media, family), that you can love yourself IF (fill in the blank). If you make a certain income, if you do x amount of good deeds a year, if you've ridden yourself of all your hidden shameful habits. And as both old and modern fairy tales still teach us, you can only love yourself once you are loved by another.

The industry of love has in many ways hijacked true love. Here is my experience of true love: it is unconditional. If I leave you with one thing to take from this book, it is this: if you make NO positive shifts in your life from this book or any other book, if nothing about you changes, you are still a being worthy of love and worthy of *your* love.

There has been a huge recent upswing in the realm of wellness and self care. And that's amazing and taps into a growing consciousness around holistic health. But here's what I also say. "Self care" in the absence of self kindness is NOT self love. There are people flogging themselves in the gym in the name of self care. If you are scolding yourself for not having been able to fit in your massage session, you are missing the entire point. And I say that with absolute kindness.

What is known by anyone who either experiences sustained positive habit change or teaches it, is that shame is never a good motivator for lasting change. It might work short term but I think at the heart of shame is self-loathing. It deals with "I am bad" not "I did bad" (Dr. Brené Brown talks about this eloquently in her work and her TED talk on this subject at the time of this writing has over 8 million views[8] which I think speaks in part to how hungry many of us are for self-love. I think there is something innate and self-loving in all of us that balks at any change which comes from a place of shame and self-loathing. We resist it hard, which is why so many people experience "yo-yo" dieting or relapse in whatever habit they are trying to release. If this is you, I invite you to look at not just what you are doing to release the habit you want to let go of, but HOW you are doing it, and specifically, how you speak to yourself about it. Especially when you relapse. I remember in the early days of healing my binge eating disorder, having such frustration with myself when I would relapse. I thought to myself, "but I know better now! I am eating healthier foods (though I still had a lot to learn, in turned out), I'm in therapy! Why is this still happening? What is wrong with me? Why am I punishing myself like this?" And these thoughts were very much accompanied with an energy of anger and disgust with myself. And it never worked. The self scolding never worked in helping me reach my goal of healing this disorder. Because what I really needed outside of the self care practice of therapy and eating healthier, was self kindness. I needed total self acceptance. I needed to know that if I never changed, if for the rest of my life I was struggling with my disordered eating behavior, I could still love myself and see myself worthy of being loved. And that was hard. It flew in the face of my perfectionism, of what I envisioned for my ideal life (and eating this way was not part of it).

So what helped me do it, to really accept myself? 3 things.

1. Understanding that it is ONLY through self acceptance that one can paradoxically make lasting *self-loving* change.
2. Understanding that something wasn't wrong with me; that at the crux of it all, I wasn't defunct or self-annihilating because of my addiction/disordered eating behavior. That actually at the heart of it, my body and soul and mind were doing all they could to take care of me. And this way of disordered eating was the way my self knew how to take care of me. In other words, I had to look past the behavior to see how the behavior was *serving* me. What was it providing for me? And as I wrote about at length in Chapter 5, my disordered eating served a very important role of self preservation in shielding me from powerful feelings that I had difficulty processing. Once I learned how to embrace and process and release those emotions, the binge eating was no longer needed. But first again, I had to understand that my bingeing behavior didn't come from an inside place of "I hate you" but rather a place of "I love you, and this is what we've got as a tool to not have you feel such pain...so here goes. But hey, um, let us know when you've got some better tools, okay?"

3. I had to practice. As part of my morning meditation, I say to myself "I love myself as I am and I am worthy of love exactly as I am." I still do it. There are too many messages in the world that carry the song of conditional love. Telling myself at least once a day that I am unconditionally loved and lovable isn't too much for me. I encourage you to start being aware of how you speak to yourself about yourself. What words do you use, what tone do you use? It can often be the case that we speak to others far more kindly and with more care than we speak to ourselves, and not only is that sad, it doesn't really last very long. Sooner or later, we start treating others (especially those closest to us) similarly to the way we treat ourselves, maybe a little better but not much. Because again, we are all connected. This step might seem not genuine at first, it might feel fake. Well I could say "practice the 'fake it till you make it' philosophy with this." But I would like to offer something other than that. The reminder that you loving yourself is actually NOT fake. That maybe you've forgotten to love yourself or how to, but as mentioned before, it's in our DNA to practice self-love and self-preservation. So if you say to yourself in the mirror, or silently after meditation or standing in the line in the grocery store or at a stoplight, "I love myself as I am and I am worthy of love exactly as I am," and you feel resistance, carry on. Keep doing it until it no longer feels uncomfortable, until you're not just saying it, you are wearing and living it.

As I mentioned before, there is a lot of input from media and music about romantic love, not surprisingly. One thing I started doing during my health journey around self-love was changing the lyrics in my head with songs that had to do with regaling the other. I'll give you a specific example. Closet song crush alert: "From This Moment On" by Shania Twain. I used to play this song in my room, singing along, usually accompanied by a fantasy of the perfect man and said perfect man and I on our wedding day. It's a great happily-ever-after song. Lyrics like "you are the one," "I live only for your happiness," "for your love, I'd give my last breath," "my dreams came true because of you," "all we need is just the two of us." All beautiful. But it kind of sucks if you're waiting on someone for your life to start. And this song is not unique on waxing poetic about an external dependency on love and life. Once I started doing the above three exercises I shared with you, this song began to make me pause. My eyes would open a sentence or two into the song with an eyebrow raise. In fact I begin giving a lot of songs the "side-eye" and it was ruining my playlists. So I started changing the lyrics. I started changing the song to "*I* am the one," "My dreams came true because of me." It didn't feel like self-obsession, it felt like self-affirmation. It felt like I was responsible and powerful enough to create a life of love and happiness and I didn't need to wait for a Prince Charming to hand it to me, for my life to begin. And ironically and probably not surprisingly, once I mastered this, the perfect man (for me) came along— a whole man practicing self love, who recognized me doing the same.

So I invite you to take a look at your music playlists, at the movies and TV shows you watch, and to just become more conscious of what you watch, listen to, read; what you take in. I still watch movies and read books about co-dependency and other unhealthy love relationship dynamics, but I do it with FAR more consciousness and awareness, and if anything, if the works are true works of art, I've found they often provide affirmation around the importance of self-love practices.

One of the more concrete ways that I saw increased self love have a hugely positive impact on my health was through minimalism. As I nurtured the above shared self-love practices along with some of the self care practices offered throughout this book, my desire for consumption decreased dramatically. I felt the need to buy and own less stuff. Specifically, for me, less books.

You see, before an awareness of my self-love (or lack there-of), I was book obsessed.

Preparing for my first departure from New York City after completing my medical residency, a very important event occurred that helped me come face-to-face with my compulsive book buying habit: I was cussed out by a trio of women in the East Village post office on Avenue A.

How did this happen? Well I happened to be in front of them in line on a sweltering July day and the post office had a broken air conditioner. Along side me were 20 (that's twenty) book boxes that I had painstakingly prepared, each packed to the brim with books of poetry, novels, novellas, plays, memoirs, biographies and of course medical books, none of which seemed appropriate to part with. I was on my way to West Africa shortly to do medical field work and carting 20 book boxes with me there was not an option. So I was shipping all of the boxes to the home of my best friend's parents who were too kind enough to keep the boxes in their attic until I figured out how to deal with them. Side note— after shipping the boxes, it took me more than 5 years to make it to that attic and reckon with all those words. So here I am alone at the height of NYC's humid summers, with 20 book boxes and trying to carry each one of them to one of the post office windows. It is taking a lot of time, and the ladies behind me are not having it. They are speaking Spanish maybe to protect me (I think not) but I understand every word and those around me who don't speak Spanish can at least understand "loca" and/or the look on the women's faces. A young guy walks into the post office, takes pity on me and starts helping me with my load. And that's when I realized, "yeah, this is a bit loca." It would take me a few years to really let go of the bulk of my possessions but I am in gratitude for that moment in the post office as my first wake up call.

Fast forward 10 years and everything I own can fit into a duffel bag, including my library card (I've never stopped loving to read). And I've never been happier or felt more at peace.

Those ten years were marked by the health journey lessons that I am sharing in this book, a key one being self-love. I look back now and see that for me, a lot of the voracious reading I was doing, was a search for the story that would help me feel better about myself. And I would get it by reading about people who were even more self-loathing than I was, or whose circumstances were so awful, that I would be soothed by my situation, even though I knew I could do better. It stoked my complacency. It was the erudite literature version of rubber-necking. And really, it was no better than those who are addicted to reality TV shows featuring people with drama-filled (and often exaggerated) messy personalities and lives. Now to be clear, I still read some of those books but like with movies, I do it now from a place of compassion, empathy and a healthy distance, not as a needy maw hungry for self-affirmation. And I think that's at the heart of it. The stuff that is crowding your life and health to the point of near suffocation might be books, clothes, video games, social media and the world wide web, or as we've already talked about before, food. Whatever it is, the compulsion to buy/consume any of these to excess often comes from a place of not being able to sit with oneself. Again, please see Chapter 5 for support with this.

I found a synergistically powerful effect in both decluttering and working on my emotion honoring release practice, bit by bit. As I decluttered, I rid myself of blocked, trapped energies that no longer served me, and that new space gave the ability for emotions to rise up to the surface to be acknowledged, embraced, and released. And conversely, as I practiced consistently acknowledging, embracing, learning from and then releasing my emotions, I felt more spacious and more centered. Furthermore, I found that as I did this practice, I wanted my home to reflect that sense of spaciousness and centeredness, Thus, I needed less things in my living space to distract me or to numb my emotions since I was finally honoring them. And though I write in the past tense, this practice is not an activity of the past. It continues. Like a seasonal nutritional detox, I also now seasonally "detox" my surroundings. And seasonally is a loose term— I do think there is transformational power in the turning of the seasons and so I definitely declutter and detox during these times. But there are also the "seasons of one's life" and I use big events in my life (a significant physical change of environment, a change in relationship) but also the small more nuanced ones like lowered energy/sluggishness, as an opportunity to declutter and simplify. During this process, I take a good look at what I have and ask myself if I love the item and also if it supports my healthiest, happiest life that I desire. And if it doesn't, I let it go with gratitude. I let it go with gratitude for it having served a purpose in my life, until now, with the acknowledgment that it's time to let it go and free up energy and space. It is a practice that I now love—detoxing my belongings and space as a physical and emotional cleanse and reset. There has been a huge increase in interest around a minimalist lifestyle during the past several years. One reason for this is financially motivated; however, for many, it is also the persistent, increasingly itchy doubt that more stuff (outside the basic requirements of shelter, food, potable water etc) doesn't translate to more health or happiness. In fact studies seems to show that the inverse is true. Now you might be a bit confused thinking— "how did this chapter get taken over by a talk on minimalism and me getting rid of stuff, I thought it was about love??" And it is. And here is what I would offer for consideration, based on my experience and those of many who have undergone the process of letting go of baggage, literally. Releasing stuff is a clear reflection and declaration of the fact that *you are enough*. To be who you are,

Dr. Tumi Johnson, M.D.

to be lovable, to be worthy of any goodness, you do not need x, y, z. And there is power in that. Releasing stuff frees up space, but not just outside of you— such as in your living space—but also within yourself. People inevitably say after decluttering, "I feel lighter," "I feel a burden lifted," because as pretty as objects x, y, z, might be, they can carry lots of weight. I believe creating space within is one of the most loving acts one can do for oneself. It is a reflection of the expansiveness that is true love itself. It is freedom. And that to me is health embodied.

I tried a bunch of things— prayer, yoga, green tea. Some of them worked, some didn't but I remember the words of my future self at the edge of my hospital bed years ago when living felt more painful than dying. *"Stay in bhujangasana longer than you care to be. Pray for what you desire, and wear color."* I am proud, humbled, and thankful to say that through much I have shared in this book, I have grown into that wild woman with poetry tucked under her arm and I lean in now and say to you as the final words to this book: just write the "song that gets you through," the song that helps you dance along life's paths.

Much much love.

My Prescription for Nurturing Self Love (three tips):

1. Say something kind to yourself every day.
2. Do something kind for yourself every day.
3. Do something kind for someone else every day.

REFERENCES

*Note: all the below Reference URLs can be found as clickable links on my website at www.drtumijohnson.com under "The Book" tab.

Chapter 1

1) McDonaldization was a term used by sociologist George Ritzer in his book The McDonaldization of Society (1993). It is described in the book as what occurs when a society takes on the qualities of a fast-food restaurants.

2) Some books, medical studies, and websites that were helpful for me and which share the health benefits of a plant foods diet:
    * Journey to Health by Annette Larkins
    * Prevent and Reverse Heart Disease by Caldwell Esselstyn MD
    * Dr. Neal Barnard's Program for Reversing Diabetes by Neal Barnard MD
    * The China Study by T Colin Campbell PhD and Thomas M Campbell II MD
    * Becoming Vegan by Brenda Davis RD, Vesanto Melina MS RD
    * The 80/10/10 Diet by Dr. Douglas Graham
    * Fruitarianism: The Path to Paradise by Anne Osbourne
    * https://www.ornish.com/wp-content/uploads/Intensive_Lifestyle_Changes_and_Prostate_Cancer.pdf
    * http://www.dresselstyn.com/site/study01/

* http://www.dresselstyn.com/Esselstyn_Three-case-reports_Exp-Clin-Cardiol-July-2014.pdf

* http://journals.plos.org/plosone/article?id=10.1371/journal.pone.0140846

* PCRM.org

* NutritionFacts.org

3) http://journals.sagepub.com/doi/abs/10.1177/0956797613478949

4) http://ajcn.nutrition.org/content/early/2013/02/25/ajcn.112.045245.abstract

5) Kristeller JL, Wolever RQ. Mindfulness-based eating awareness training for treating binge eating disorder: the conceptual foundation. Eat Disord. 2011;19(1): 49-61.

6) Daubenmier J, Kristeller J, Hecht FM, et al. Mindfulness intervention for stress eating to reduce cortisol and abdominal fat among overweight and obese women: an exploratory randomized controlled study. J Obes. 2011; 2011: 651936.

7) Timmerman GM, Brown A. The effect of a mindful restaurant eating intervention on weight management in women. J Nutr Educ Behav. 2012;44(1):22-28.

Chapter 2

1) http://www.ajpmonline.org/article/S0749-3797(16)00048-9/fulltext http://performinghealing.com/en-US/a-155675/posture-back-pain-neck-paincervicalgia-life-expectancy-mindfulness

2) http://onlinelibrary.wiley.com/doi/10.1111/aphw.12058/abstract?campaign=woletoc

3) Auvinen J., Tammelin T., Taimela S., Zitting P., Karppinen J. Neck and shoulder pains in relation to physical activity and sedentary activities in adolescence. Spine. 2007;32(9):1038–1044. [PubMed]

4) https://www.ncbi.nlm.nih.gov/pmc/articles/PMC2528269/

5) http://www.ajpmonline.org/article/S0749-3797(16)00048-9/fulltext

6) http://standing-desk.sqwiz.com/

Chapter 3

1) http://archinte.jamanetwork.com/article.aspx?articleid=1809754

2) http://onlinelibrary.wiley.com/doi/10.1002/jts.21936/full

3) http://www.ncbi.nlm.nih.gov/pmc/articles/PMC4437062/

4) http://pss.sagepub.com/content/24/9/1714

5) https://www.drweil.com/weekly-bulletin/the-relaxation-response/

Chapter 4

1) https://www.ncbi.nlm.nih.gov/pmc/articles/PMC2864873/

2) https://www.ncbi.nlm.nih.gov/pubmed/26118561

3) Knutson KL, et al. Role of Sleep Duration and Quality in the Risk and Severity of Type 2 Diabetes Mellitus, Archives of Internal Medicine. 2006 Sep 18; 166(16):1768.
https://www.ncbi.nlm.nih.gov/pubmed/16983057

4) Gottlieb DJ, et al. Association of Sleep Time with Diabetes Mellitus and Impaired Glucose Tolerance, Archives of Internal Medicine. 2005 Apr 25; 165(8): 863. https://www.ncbi.nlm.nih.gov/pubmed/15851636

5) https://www.ncbi.nlm.nih.gov/pubmed/27804960

6) https://www.nih.gov/news-events/nih-research-matters/molecular -ties-between-lack-sleep-weight-gain

7) https://www.ncbi.nlm.nih.gov/pmc/articles/PMC4318605/

8) https://www.ncbi.nlm.nih.gov/pubmed/15680291

9) King, CR et al. Short Sleep Duration and Incident Coronary Artery Calcification, JAMA, 2008: 300(24): 2859-2866 https://www.ncbi.nlm.nih.gov/pubmed/19109114

10) Spiegel K, et al. Impact of Sleep Debt on Metabolic and Endocrine Function, Lancet. 1999 Oct 23: 354(9188): 1435-9. https://www.ncbi.nlm.nih.gov/pubmed/10543671

11) https://www.cdc.gov/features/dsdrowsydriving/index.html

12) http://jamanetwork.com/journals/jama/fullarticle/2516715?utm_source =TWITTER&utm_medium=social_jn&utm_term=4480390 38&utm_content=content_engagement|article_engagement&utm _campaign=press_release&linkId=23887023

13) https://www.healio.com/~/media/Journals/AAOHN/2012/5 _May/10_3928_21650799_20120416_22/10_3928_21650799_20120 416_22.ashx

14) https://www.ncbi.nlm.nih.gov/pubmed/9891131

15) http://stm.sciencemag.org/content/4/129/129ra43

16) https://www.ncbi.nlm.nih.gov/pmc/articles/PMC4538113/

17) http://journals.plos.org/plosone/article?id=10.1371/journal. pone.0020708

18) http://www.sciencedirect.com/science/article/pii/S0022103113002205

19) http://www.tandfonline.com/doi/abs/10.1080/10400419.2014. 901073#preview

20) https://www.ncbi.nlm.nih.gov/pubmed/15507147/

21) http://www.wombblessing.com/eng-books.html Miranda Gray Female Energy Awakening

Chapter 5

1) http://www.veronicakrestow.com/audio-flip-book/

Chapter 6

1) http://journals.sagepub.com/doi/abs/10.1111/j.1467-9280.2008.02225.x

2) http://www.sciencedirect.com/science/article/pii/S0165032712002005

3) https://www.ncbi.nlm.nih.gov/pmc/articles/PMC5551166/

4) https://www.ncbi.nlm.nih.gov/pubmed/20337470

5) https://www.ncbi.nlm.nih.gov/pmc/articles/PMC2793347/

6) https://www.ncbi.nlm.nih.gov/pubmed/26124129

7) https://www.ncbi.nlm.nih.gov/pmc/articles/PMC1448497/

8) http://journals.sagepub.com/doi/abs/10.1177/1087054708323000

9) https://www.ncbi.nlm.nih.gov/pubmed/18394317

10) https://www.ncbi.nlm.nih.gov/pmc/articles/PMC2793346/

11) https://www.ncbi.nlm.nih.gov/pubmed/21996763

12) https://www.ted.com/talks/ron_finley_a_guerilla_gardener_in_south_central_la

Chapter 7

[1] https://www.ncbi.nlm.nih.gov/pubmed/25243717

[2] http://self-compassion.org/

[3] https://www.ncbi.nlm.nih.gov/pubmed/22282874

[4] https://www.ncbi.nlm.nih.gov/pubmed/16905215

[5] https://www.ncbi.nlm.nih.gov/pubmed/22021599

ACKNOWLEDGMENTS

I give thanks first to Spirit, to the great I Am who whispered the calling to write this book into my ear one day during meditation. The still small Voice that has guided my steps always, even when I was unaware of it.

I thank my parents— my mother who increasingly embodies joy, and my father who told me always to keep my head high. I thank my sisters Lola and Tola, who have blessed my life with laughter, love, beauty, and that special bond that only sisters who have navigated childhood together, share.

I thank my friends who though are scattered throughout the globe, are my tribe. You know who you are and I am grateful for your love and your nourishing friendship. I would especially like to thank here the first readers of an excerpt of this book. Thank you for holding with kindness, space for me to share myself vulnerably and authentically: Andrea Truncali, Alka Khaitan, Carrie Mahowald, and Sharon Lerner.

I thank Balboa Press and Hay House Publishing for giving me the opportunity to share this book with others.

And to Zarko Manojlovič— my adventure partner and beloved sweetheart. Thank you for your unwavering encouragement and support during the creation of this book, and for sharing this delicious life with me.

To connect with me,
you can find me on
Instagram: thepoemdances
You Tube: thepoemdances

For more on my holistic medical practice,
please visit: www.drtumijohnson.com
For more on my dance work, please check
out: www.tumijohnson.com

Much love to you.